INTERNATIONAL DEVELOPMENT IN PRACTICE

Planning National Telemedicine and Health Hotline Services

A Toolkit for Governments

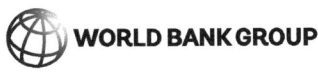
WORLD BANK GROUP

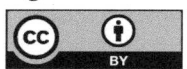

Contents

Acknowledgments

This toolkit was produced by the World Bank in collaboration with the Ministry of Health of Libya. It is an output of the Libya Health Sector Support Grant (P163565) program led by Christopher H. Herbst and Mohini Kak, both senior health specialists at the World Bank.

Carla Blauvelt of VillageReach prepared this toolkit with contributions from Brandon Bowersox-Johnson, Upile Kachila, Amanda Pain, Jennifer Pancholi, Joseph Roussel, Steven Simkonda, and Anderson Ti-Timi, and from Derek Ritz of ecGroup Inc. Joaquin Blaya (consultant, World Bank) oversaw the technical development of the report, with inputs from Christopher H. Herbst and Mohini Kak. The team thanks two of the contributors of the Pan American Health Organization/World Health Organization *Framework for the Implementation of a Telemedicine Service*—Marcelo D'Agostino and Francesc Saigí Rubió—for initial discussions and inputs, as well as peer reviewers Matthew Thomas Hulse and Zlatan Sabic from the World Bank for valuable inputs and feedback that helped improve the quality of the report.

Glossary

This toolkit uses the terms *telehealth* and *telemedicine* interchangeably, as they are used in peer-reviewed work.

Telehealth or **telemedicine:**

Delivery of health care services, where patients and providers are separated by distance. Telehealth uses ICT (information and communications technology) for the exchange of information for the diagnosis and treatment of diseases and injuries, research, and evaluation, and for the continuing education of health professionals. Telehealth can contribute to achieving universal health coverage by improving access for patients to quality, cost-effective, health services wherever they may be. It is particularly valuable for those in remote areas, vulnerable groups and ageing populations. (WHO 2016)

Health hotline: A continuously managed telephone or communication line for individuals to communicate with professionals who answer questions about general health or disease or provide resources for individuals experiencing crises (impending suicide, poisoning, domestic violence, rape, drugs, among others) (O'Toole 2005).

Solution: The *what* needed and the *how* required to solve a defined problem. The components that make up a solution can include a combination of processes, products, principles, organization, tools, metrics, and collaboration that provides the functionalities needed to solve a defined problem. For the purposes of this toolkit, the solution we are discussing is the combination of elements that make up the government's chosen telemedicine or health hotline services (VillageReach 2021).

Service provider: A vendor that provides solutions or services to end users and organizations.[1] For the purposes of this toolkit, such vendors could be mobile network operators, organizations providing telemedicine or health hotline services, or organizations providing technical software or additive elements (WhatsApp, interactive voice response, and so on).

Low- and middle-income countries: Countries defined as such by the World Bank Group (https://datahelpdesk.worldbank.org/knowledgebase/articles /906519). Because this toolkit aims to help governments implementing a national-scale system, it focuses on countries with a central health ministry that makes decisions for a public health system and reflects the processes and timelines with which those organizations work.

NOTE

1. See https://www.techopedia.com/definition/22021/service-provider.

REFERENCES

O'Toole, M., ed. 2005. *Miller-Keane Encyclopedia & Dictionary of Medicine, Nursing & Allied Health*, 7th edition. London: Saunders.

VillageReach. 2021. "Journey to Scale with Government: The Mindset Shift." https://www .villagereach.org/wp-content/uploads/2020/10/The-Journey-to-Scale-with-Government -Interactive-Tool_Final-2.pdf.

WHO (World Health Organization). 2016. *Global Diffusion of eHealth: Making Universal Health Coverage Achieveable*. Geneva: World Health Organization. https://apps.who.int/iris/rest /bitstreams/1071614/retrieve.

Main Messages

The coronavirus (COVID-19) pandemic has illustrated that many countries still lack the necessary primary health care system to support their populations, as well as efficient ways to quickly disperse and collect health information. Although many countries worked with local mobile network operators and other partners to assist with immediate COVID-19 information and reporting needs, governments throughout the world, regardless of economic status, have identified the need for robust digital health care solutions. Telemedicine or health hotline services allow people to receive accurate and timely health information, and to make informed decisions on when to seek treatment. The ability to provide health information and care remotely also reduces the number of patients that health workers see in person, which increases those workers' capacity to serve their communities. These services therefore extend the reach of the health care system, improve efficiencies in it, and enhance the quality of care it provides (PAHO 2016).

Health services that are stewarded by government and embedded into public health systems, are more likely to sustain impact at scale. Despite telemedicine's demonstrated positive impact for more than 60 years, few nationally scaled telemedicine or health hotline services exist—and even fewer are government owned. Many digital health solutions are set up for emergency response or with donor funding but are never embedded within the government systems and budgets. Many solutions fail, despite effectiveness or impact, because they were developed without government input and without a plan for government to eventually steward the solution. This toolkit builds on existing evidence to help governments establish successful nationwide telemedicine or health hotline services.

For the success of national-scale telemedicine and hotline services, governments must work through the following three major phases.

First, governments must assess basic requirements and expressions of interest. This phase entails an assessment of whether a telemedicine or hotline service aligns with government policy, and an assessment of political stability in the country—that is, does reliable support exist for what may be a long-term initiative? Assuming political stability and alignment with policy, the government must look at technical considerations. For example, assessing available infrastructure, including power and connectivity in the country, will allow the government to understand the level of readiness for the setup and effective use of telemedicine services. Finally, the government must express interest in launching the service and dedicate human resources toward further exploration.

Second, governments must scope and design the solution. This phase entails designating a focal point, setting up a task force, and identifying the roles of various departments and partners that would be involved in setting up and scaling the system. Following that organizational step, governments must scope out the actual solution—that is, determining which areas of the health system the service will address and who the target audience will be, estimating uptake, and conducting a landscape analysis to understand the relevant resources already available in the country. Finally, the task force must actually design the solution, taking into account the findings of the various scoping activities.

Third, governments must develop a strategy, an implementation road map, and a budget. This phase entails first establishing a multisector steering committee to develop a five-year strategic plan for setting up and maintaining the telemedicine service. That plan will include solution management, impact or outcome, health areas covered, specific services provided, and geographic coverage. The steering committee would have responsibility for signing off on the scope defined by the task force, assuming it aligns with the strategic plan. Further, the government must ensure that it has a plan for engaging with the private sector—including, among others, telemedicine service providers and mobile network operators. All key stakeholders in government must be involved in developing this engagement strategy and should ensure that the government remains the steward of the solution. This step also involves working with mobile network operations to set up short codes and zero-rate calls. Next, the government must develop a one-year implementation plan and identify the appropriate technologies and partners for implementation of a secure, sustainable, well-staffed, and effective solution that fits into the overall health information landscape of the country, taking into account interoperability, data privacy, and any infrastructure constraints. Finally, the strategy and the implementation road map need to be costed out and validated, and requests for proposals drafted and issued so that service providers can place their bids.

Carefully considering and addressing all three areas and their nuances and specifics as detailed in this toolkit is critical for positioning the government and its partners to set up and run a successful national-scale telemedicine service.

REFERENCE

PAHO (Pan American Health Organization). 2016. *Framework for the Implementation of a Telemedicine Service.* Washington, DC: PAHO. https://iris.paho.org/bitstream/handle /10665.2/28414/9789275119037_eng.pdf?sequence=6&isAllowed=y.

Abbreviations

CCPF   Chipatala Cha Pa Foni
COVID-19   coronavirus
IT   information technology
M&E   monitoring and evaluation
MNO   mobile network operator
RFP   request for proposal
RFQ   request for quotation
SMS   Short Message Service
TOR   terms of reference

Overview

For many low- and middle-income countries, telemedicine and health hotlines are the best way to increase community access to health information and health care. The importance of this type of service became even more apparent during the coronavirus pandemic, when countries with low ratios of health care workers to population—and large populations living far from a health center—needed better ways for their citizens to access health information and care. In many countries, telemedicine and health hotline services have played an important role in filling these access gaps. Ensuring the national-scale impact of such services, however, requires involving the government from the beginning and having a longer-term plan for government stewardship of the solution.

For a solution to be sustainable, it must be incorporated into country strategies and budgets, and the government must have ownership of the solution even if it outsources all or parts of the operation. Although there are several ways to set up telemedicine and health hotline services, this toolkit is based on VillageReach's experiences with governments in the Democratic Republic of Congo, Kenya, Malawi, and Mozambique, including its work with the Malawi Ministry of Health to establish one of Sub-Saharan Africa's first government-owned nationwide health hotline services—Chipatala Cha Pa Foni, or Health Center by Phone (https://www.youtube.com/watch?v=hzPR8A3yQc4).

This toolkit focuses on health hotlines and telemedicine, specifically on the telemedicine systems used for primary care services rather than for specialized care, such as tele-dermatology, tele-oncology, and others. Building on the Pan American Health Organization/World Health Organization *Framework for the Implementation of a Telemedicine Service* (https://iris.paho.org/bitstream/handle /10665.2/28414/9789275119037_eng.pdf?sequence=6&isAllowed=y), the toolkit is intended for use by high-level government officials and technical teams setting up national-scale telemedicine or health hotline services in their country (PAHO 2016). It outlines the multiphased approach needed to set up a health hotline or telemedicine service at a national scale and provides tools that can be used to, for example, cost out and design the system, contract service providers, and engage mobile network operators. That approach involves the following phases: (0) assess basic requirements and express interest; (1) scope and design the solution; (2) develop strategy, implementation road map, and budget solution;

(3) secure funding for the start-up period; and (4) establish, implement, scale, and sustain the solution. Because activities in Phases 3 and 4 will be very specific to the context of a country and the chosen solution, this toolkit does not cover them. It details the activities in Phases 0–2 in three sections that outline the following activities by phase.

- **Phase 0: Assess basic requirements and express interest**
    - Assess the basic political stability requirements.
    - Review the minimum technology considerations.
    - Express interest and commitment to devote human resource time for further exploration.
- **Phase 1: Scope and design solution**
    - Establish a focal point and small planning task force within the government.
    - Understand the necessary stakeholder champions required for sustained impact at scale.
    - Determine what audience and health topics should be addressed with a telemedicine or health hotline service given the specific country context.
    - Assess available resources in-country that the government can leverage.
    - Develop a high-level functional solution design for planning and costing in Phase 2.
- **Phase 2: Develop strategy, implementation road map, and budget solution**
    - Establish a cross-sectoral decision-making steering committee.
    - Develop a five-year sustainability strategy.
    - Develop a private sector strategy.
    - Set up the one-year road map for implementation.
    - Develop the terms of reference to select the best combination of technologies.
    - Estimate preliminary costs for the five-year strategy and one-year road map.
    - Define the immediate next steps for the government to establish services.

During **Phase 0**, the government must investigate whether a telemedicine or health hotline service could be successful and sustainable. It does so by assessing the basic level of political stability, whether the proposed service aligns with current government priorities, and whether the country has the technical readiness to launch this solution—for example, by looking at the level of cell phone use and internet access. Having assessed these factors, and if the government decides to proceed on the basis of the results, it should move on to Phase 1.

During **Phase 1**, the government should establish a planning task force and focal point within the ministry of health to identify key stakeholders and make critical decisions on the target audience, potential health topics, and potential community and health worker uptake. During this phase, the government will require a needs assessment, a landscape analysis, and an uptake assessment. Once it has completed these activities, and if the planning task force recommends moving forward, the government can move to Phase 2.

Phase 2 outlines how the government will establish a decision-making body, such as a steering committee, to align with the vision for the service; make a preliminary plan for implementation; and determine the cost of the proposed solution, strategy, and road map. These steps are critical to helping ensure, from the outset, the solution's sustainability. This toolkit includes five chapters to guide the government in creating and validating a five-year strategy (chapter 5); developing a private sector strategy, because the technology needed will likely require a private sector partner (chapter 6); developing a one-year road map for implementation planning (chapter 7); selecting the best technologies and partners for a sustainable, integrated solution (chapter 8); and costing the solution, strategy, and road map (chapter 9).

Despite the number of activities recommended, it is still possible to establish a telemedicine or health hotline service in 3–12 months, depending on the level of government commitment, available service providers, and available financial resources in the country. One of the best ways for governments to learn about best practices, challenges, and sustainable approaches to establishing telemedicine or health hotline services is to talk to other governments that have gone through the process. Additionally, interested governments will find it incredibly valuable to visit any existing service centers to see how they are managed.

REFERENCE

PAHO (Pan American Health Organization). 2016. *Framework for the Implementation of a Telemedicine Service*. Washington, DC: PAHO. https://iris.paho.org/bitstream/handle /10665.2/28414/9789275119037_eng.pdf?sequence=6&isAllowed=y.

Introduction

BENEFITS OF TELEMEDICINE OR HEALTH HOTLINE SERVICES

The COVID-19 pandemic has illustrated that many countries still lack the necessary primary health care system to support their populations, as well as efficient ways to quickly disperse and collect health information. Although many countries worked with local mobile network operators and other partners to assist with immediate COVID-19 information and reporting needs, governments throughout the world, regardless of economic status, have identified the need for robust digital health care solutions. Telemedicine or health hotline services allow people to receive accurate and timely health information, and to make informed decisions on when to seek treatment. The ability to provide health information or care remotely also reduces the number of patients health workers see in person, which increases these workers' capacity to serve their communities. These services therefore extend the reach of the health care system, improve efficiencies in it, and enhance the quality of care it provides (PAHO 2016).

Health services that are stewarded by government and embedded into public health systems are more likely to sustain impact at scale. Despite telemedicine's demonstrated positive impact for more than 60 years, few nationally scaled telemedicine or health hotline services exist—and even fewer are government owned. Many digital health solutions are set up for emergency response or with donor funding but are never embedded within government systems and budgets. Development of these solutions without government input and without a plan for government to eventually steward the solution often leads to their failure, despite effectiveness or impact.

This toolkit builds on existing evidence to help governments establish successful nationwide telemedicine or health hotline services. Although telemedicine or health hotline services can be set up quickly, the steps included in this toolkit are for governments committed to having long-term, sustainable services embedded in the public health system.

This toolkit builds on the Pan American Health Organization/World Health Organization *Framework for the Implementation of a Telemedicine Service* (https://iris.paho.org/bitstream/handle/10665.2/28414/9789275119037_eng .pdf?sequence=6&isAllowed=y), which provides a theoretical framework for successfully implementing telemedicine services in a country (PAHO 2016). That framework can be read before using this toolkit, which then provides the actionable tools needed to plan and implement services. The toolkit also builds on VillageReach's experience working with governments to establish these services in three countries—the Democratic Republic of Congo, Kenya, Malawi, and Mozambique. For example, in Malawi, VillageReach codeveloped, established, and transitioned Chipatala Cha Pa Foni (CCPF), or Health Center by Phone (https://www.youtube.com/watch?v=hzPR8A3yQc4), with the Ministry of Health (VillageReach 2019). CCPF is a free nationwide health hotline and messaging service that has been correlated with increased knowledge and health behaviors (https://www.villagereach.org/wp-content/uploads/2020/02/VR _CCPFImpactEval_FINAL.-2_24_20-1.pdf)—see figure 1.1 (VillageReach 2019, 2020). The Malawi government added CCPF to its health sector strategic plans and budgets, ensuring its sustainability. Having this service in place also allowed the government to quickly adapt CCPF for its COVID-19 response, which experienced a call volume increase of 542 percent from February 2020 to March 2021. Figure 1.2 shows the geographic scope, health topics, and cost of CCPF over time. The increase in costs from 2017 to 2019 resulted from technology upgrades and expansion nationwide. Once the technology upgrades were complete, the ongoing maintenance costs greatly reduced and were taken on by the government.

FIGURE 1.1

Demonstrated impact of Malawi's Chipatala Cha Pa Foni, 2018

Malawi 2018

15 min
Average call time

38%
Calls made by adolescents and young adults ages 15–24

27%
Calls that lead to enrollment in Tips and Reminders

98%
CCPF user satisfaction rating of good or very good

75%
of CCPF users started ANC in their first trimester

95%
of children of CCPF users had been vaccinated or received vitamin A at least once before the survey

92%
of CCPF users were more likely to have been tested for HIV in the prior 24 months

88%
of CCPF users referred to health facilities reported going

Source: Original figure developed for this publication.
Note: Chipatala Cha Pa Foni (CCPF) is also known as Health Center by Phone. ANC = antenatal care.

FIGURE 1.2

Malawi's Chipatala Cha Pa Foni geographic scope, health topics, and costs from inception through government ownership

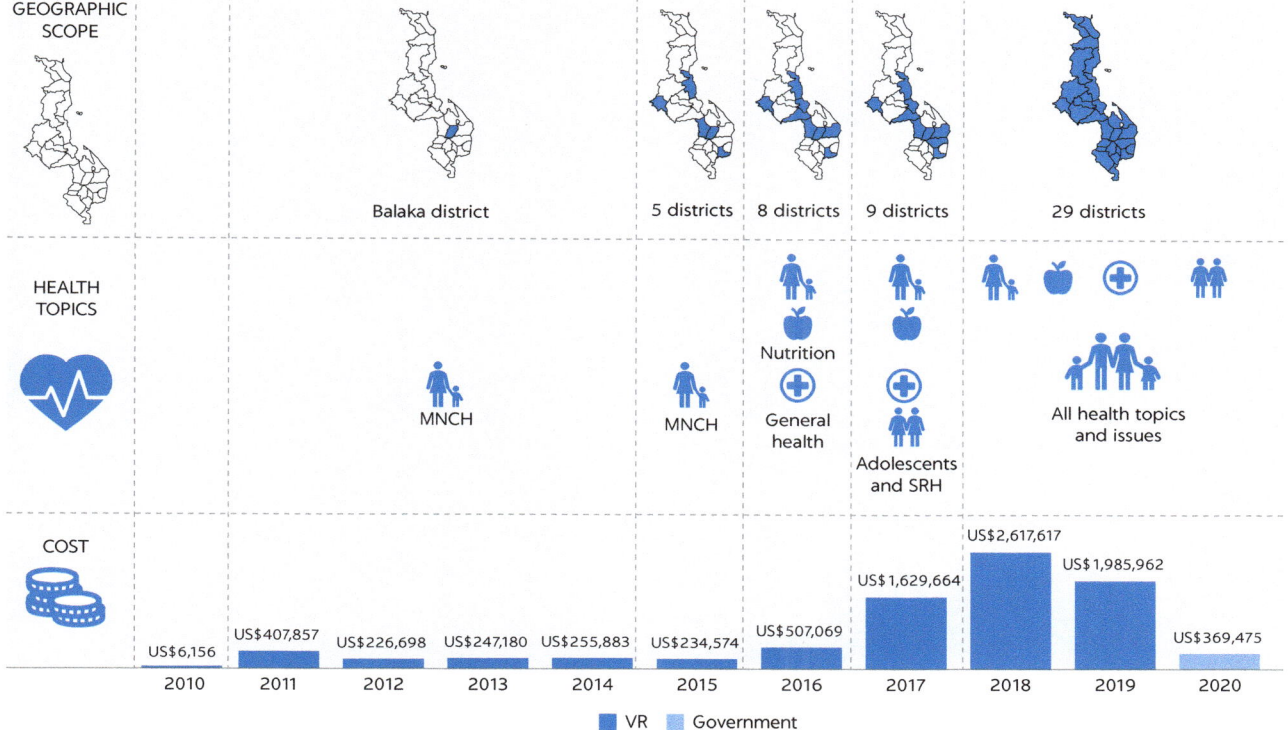

Source: Original figure developed for this publication.
Note: Chipatala Cha Pa Foni is also known as the Health Center by Phone. MNCH = maternal, newborn, and child health; SRH = sexual and reproductive health; VR = VillageReach.

PURPOSE AND SCOPE

This toolkit provides governments in low- and middle-income countries with hands-on tools to develop a strategy, a plan, and a design for nationwide telemedicine or health hotline services. It will position governments for both immediate implementation and long-term sustainability and is intended for solutions that directly serve the public through telemedicine and combined health hotline and messaging services. In addition, it offers insights into the benefits of solutions that serve members of the health workforce.

Figure 1.3 outlines the five-phase process for implementing and transitioning telemedicine or health hotline services. This toolkit is designed to assist government users from Phase 0 to Phase 2; it does not cover activities in Phases 3 and 4, because they will be very specific to the context of a country and the chosen solution. Although establishing telemedicine or health hotline services does not require all the steps in this toolkit, completing them is highly recommended. *The authors recognize that the steps in this toolkit are not the only way to achieve success and therefore offer other options for readers highlighted in the endnotes.*

FIGURE 1.3

Phases of telemedicine and health hotline planning and implementation

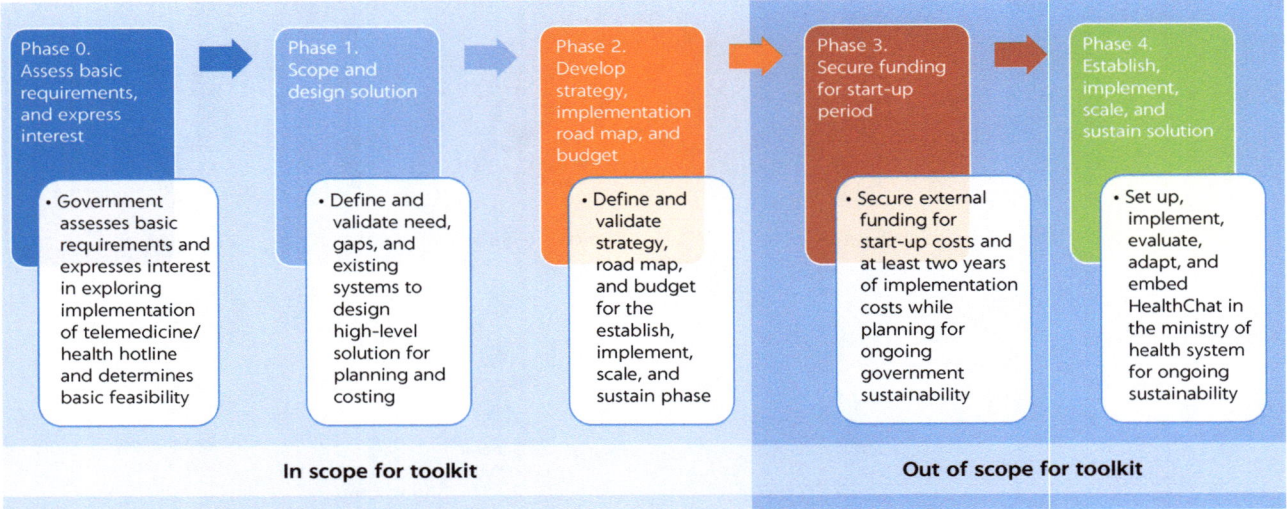

Source: Original figure developed for this publication.

Within each phase, the government will learn how to do the following:

- **Phase 0: Assess basic requirements and express interest**
  - Assess the basic political stability requirements.
  - Review the minimum technology considerations.
  - Express interest and commitment to devote human resource time for further exploration.
- **Phase 1: Scope and design the solution**
  - Establish a focal point and small planning task force within the government.
  - Understand the necessary stakeholder champions required to set the service up for sustainable impact at scale.
  - Determine what audience and health topics should be addressed with a telemedicine or health hotline service given the specific country context.
  - Assess available resources in-country that the government can leverage.
  - Develop a high-level functional solution design for planning and costing in Phase 2.
- **Phase 2: Develop strategy, implementation road map, and budget solution**
  - Establish a cross-sectoral decision-making steering committee.
  - Develop a five-year sustainability strategy.
  - Develop a private sector strategy.
  - Set up the one-year road map for implementation.
  - Develop the terms of reference to select the best combination of technologies.

- Estimate preliminary costs for the five-year strategy and one-year road map.
- Define the immediate next steps for the government to establish services.

The timeline for establishing telemedicine or hotline services will vary but will range between 3 and 12 months. A government-stewarded telemedicine or health hotline service could be established in 3–6 months for a specific health topic, like coronavirus, if existing private sector call centers are available and the necessary government approvals are met. For more extensive services that cover a range of health topics, however, establishing the service can take 6 months for existing technologies, if the approvals and validations from the government can be done quickly, or within 9–12 months if the government chooses local software companies that do not already have the needed technology. Despite the ability to quickly set up these services, it is important that governments work on a five-year strategy from the beginning to ensure sustainable impact at scale.[1]

INTENDED AUDIENCE

This toolkit is designed for high-level government officials and technical teams setting up national-scale telemedicine or health hotline services in their country. The overview sections can help high-level national government officials (directors of departments or senior management at ministries of health) determine how to approach setting up these services, and how to work toward embedding them within the public sector. The tools can be used by the technical and programmatic teams assigned to set up, plan, and eventually implement or oversee the services.

HOW TO USE THE TOOLKIT

This toolkit goes through the practical steps to plan for national-scale services and provides tools for guidance. It has three sections, with activities, milestones, and tools (if applicable) outlined in subsections. Available tools and other reference materials are underlined and linked throughout the toolkit and presented in annexes at the end of each corresponding chapter. Figure 1.4 shows the interconnection between the phases and related tools in this document.

The toolkit also includes five appendixes:

- Appendix A. Checklist of Challenges and Pitfalls That May Arise during Planning or Implementing Telemedicine or Health Hotline Services and the Mitigating Factors
- Appendix B. PowerPoint Template for Pitching Telemedicine or Health Hotline Services to Government
- Appendix C. VillageReach and Praekelt.org Sample Health Hotline and Messaging Service Pitch to a Ministry of Health
- Appendix D. Sample Implementation Toolkit from Malawi's Chipatala Cha Pa Foni
- Appendix E. Understanding Regulatory Prerequisites Reference Materials

National-scale system's real-world impact: Hawa's story

Hawa, age 20, rested in the recovery room of a district hospital in Balaka, Malawi. She had been living with a fistula for nearly three years after complications from obstructed labor while giving birth to her first child led to a C-section and a stillborn baby. Hawa was in labor for three days at her local health center, unable to deliver. Hawa's fistula condition isolated her from her community. Her husband left her, and she felt very alone. "When you have a fistula, you are stigmatized," Hawa said, looking at the floor.

Then, one day she received a text message that would change her life. It was from Chipatala Cha Pa Foni (CCPF), or Health Center by Phone. CCPF, a health hotline and message service originally run by VillageReach in partnership with Airtel and the Malawi Ministry of Health, is now operated and owned by the government. CCPF connected her with a fistula repair clinic and arranged for her transportation to the clinic for the surgery.

Hawa had her fistula surgery on October 14, 2017, at the Fistula Care Center at Bwaila District Hospital. After hearing of her story, more women have called CCPF looking for help with fistulas. CCPF has connected them with the Bwaila Fistula Foundation so that Hawa and many others now have access to the health information they need when they need it.

The private sector plays a critical role in CCPF and played a critical role in this success story. The service has always been free to users, with donors paying for the cost of the calls—and that cost was not sustainable for the government to take on long term. The government contracted with Airtel, which made calls free and provided the short code and free monthly advertising for the service to expand nationwide. Additionally, VillageReach and the Malawi Ministry of Health partnered with technology software providers to build out the hotline software. During the nationwide upgrades, VillageReach and the Ministry of Health worked with Viamo to replace and improve upon the existing software. The government now directly contracts with Viamo for ongoing system maintenance at a reduced cost and has a standing memorandum of understanding with Airtel. Airtel has also benefited from its role in CCPF because the increased number of callers to the hotline led to a request for new cell phone towers in areas that previously had low coverage.

FIGURE 1.4

Interconnection between telemedicine or health hotline phases and related tools

Entry: Government expresses preliminary interest or need

Minimum political and policy requirements tool

Minimal technical considerations checklist

Exit/entry: minimum requirements met

Terms of reference for planning task force

Stakeholder matrix

Predesign scoping tool

Private sector strategy worksheet

Five-year strategy tool

Terms of reference for steering committee

Exit/entry: solution design drafted

Solution design decision-making tool

Landscape analysis tool

Uptake assessment tool

One-year road map

Overall technical considerations checklist

Terms of reference development checklist

Selection criteria matrix

Cost model tool

Implementation and planning for sustainability from the outset checklist

Phase 3/4

Key
- Phase 0: National government expresses interest
- Phase 1: Scope and design solution
- Phase 2: Develop strategy, implementation road map, and budget

Tool

Source: Original figure developed for this publication.

NOTE

1. Although the main intention of this toolkit is not to support ongoing implementations, because that support would depend on the type of technologies and services chosen (in-house or out), some of the sections may still be useful. For example, the toolkit from Malawi's CCPF includes extensive standard operating procedures used in Malawi and adapted for Mozambique. These standard operating procedures, for combined health hotlines and messaging services, can be adapted to fit a wide range of contexts.

REFERENCES

PAHO (Pan American Health Organization). 2016. *Framework for the Implementation of a Telemedicine Service.* Washington, DC: PAHO. https://iris.paho.org/bitstream/handle/10665.2/28414/9789275119037_eng.pdf?sequence=6&isAllowed=y.

VillageReach. 2019. "Chipatala cha pa Foni (Health Center by Phone) – A Health Center in Every Malawian's Home." YouTube, June 20, 2019. https://www.youtube.com/watch?v=hzPR8A3yQc4.

VillageReach. 2020. "Impact Evaluation of Chipatala cha pa Foni (CCPF), Malawi's Health and Nutrition Hotline." Lilongwe, VillageReach Malawi. https://www.villagereach.org/wp-content/uploads/2020/02/VR_CCPFImpactEval_FINAL.-2_24_20-1.pdf.

Assess Basic Requirements and Express Interest

The prerequisite for exploring telemedicine or health hotline services is that the high-level officials in the ministry of health have assessed the basic political stability and minimum technology considerations to plan for, implement, and sustain these services. Additionally, these officials should have expressed formal, written commitment to establishing the service.

Assess Basic Political Requirements and Technical Considerations, and Express Interest

Chapter 2 helps governments consider the feasibility of telemedicine or health hotline services. It presents two tools:

- *Minimum Political and Policy Requirements Tool (annex 2A)*
- *Minimum Technical Considerations Checklist (annex 2B)*

ASSESS MINIMUM POLITICAL AND POLICY REQUIREMENTS

The sustainability of any solution requires a basic level of political stability[1] as well as ensuring that a telemedicine or health hotline service aligns with current government priorities. Even if the political will exists in the design phase and private sector partners are secured, long-term government investment of time and resources is critical to sustaining any solution impact. To assess the level of political stability, and the level of solution alignment with government policy and priorities, governments should use the tool shown in table 2.1 and annex 2A.

The questions on stability and alignment provide an initial check before developing services. Specific health policy, strategic planning, and regulatory alignment will occur later in the solution design process. If the government can answer yes for stability, it can then move forward and think through alignment with government policy and priorities. If the government answers no for stability, pursuing the services at this time would likely not be a good use of resources. The government can continue to address the political alignment, which can help it think through solution targeting—that is, who the solution audience will be and what health topics should be covered.

TABLE 2.1 Minimum political and policy requirements tool

CATEGORY	QUESTION	REASON FOR QUESTION	ANSWER
Stability	Does the government currently have basic-level political stability (that is, is it stable and functioning to meet basic needs, or is there ongoing conflict)?	Needed to ensure decision-making and leadership for establishment of the service	
	Does the government expect a basic level of stability for at least two years (that is, are there upcoming elections or anticipated political changes that would affect solution champions)?	Needed to ensure continuity in solution leadership when implementing and embedding the services into the health system	
Political alignment	Does the proposed solution align with government policy? What types of services are allowed? Will the government approve a telemedicine service designed to diagnose and treat?	Needed to ensure solution is allowed at the most basic level before it can be included in strategies and budgets and have government champions	
	Do avenues exist for ensuring that prioritized activities, such as telemedicine or health hotline services, can be financed through the government, both initially and in the long term?	Needed to ensure solution inclusion in budgets	
	Does the government have at least one focal high-level champion who will advocate for the solution to move forward?	Needed to ensure drive from the government	
	Does the proposed solution align with government priorities (investment and target geographies and beneficiaries)?	Needed to ensure solution inclusion in strategies and budgets, as well as to build government champions (Note: If the target geographies and beneficiaries the service will serve are already identified as priority areas and groups, it will be easier to make the case for the services.)	

Source: Original table developed for this publication.

ASSESS MINIMAL TECHNICAL CONSIDERATIONS FOR TELEMEDICINE OR HEALTH HOTLINE SERVICES

In addition to ensuring the solution aligns with government policy and priorities, the government also needs to understand the country's technical readiness for launching the service. The Minimum Technical Considerations Checklist in annex 2B provides governments with the basic technical requirements needed for telemedicine or health hotline services.

The main prerequisites to consider are the following:

- Information technology (IT) infrastructure for audio versus visual consultations:
  - Internet connectivity
  - Access to electricity
- Penetration of cell phone use and cell phone type

In terms of technical prerequisites, IT infrastructure is important when considering how to support audio conversations versus visual consultations. Internet connectivity and access to electricity, in terms of both geographic availability and regularity, are also important. Solutions that provide information or consultations via cell phone will depend on basic cell phone penetration or smartphone penetration.[2] The number of internet subscribers or of mobile phone subscribers offers a good proxy for measuring IT penetration if the percentage of the population owning cell phones/smartphones is unknown. Patterns in cell phone ownership, where known, can also be compared with the target groups for telemedicine and smartphone services to understand where communities may lack access to the service. Telemedicine using images or video consultations will require internet and smartphone penetration, whereas health hotlines or basic telemedicine consultations can operate with basic cell phones. When analyzing cell phone penetration, it is also important to consider the norm around shared cell phone use. For example, although in 2017 Malawi had basic cell phone penetration of 29.7 percent and smartphone penetration of 10.2 percent (Handforth and Wilson 2019), the shared use of phones among families, friends, and communities has led to increased access to the country's Chipatala Cha Pa Foni, or Health Center by Phone.

The ministry of health, in consultation with the ministry of communication, should review the considerations of IT infrastructure at an existing forum. Having data, like those available from GSMA Intelligence (https://data .gsmaintelligence.com/signin?returnPath=%2Fdata%2Fcustom-metrics -search) or documented in needs assessments, will be important for guiding discussion. (Note: You will need to create an account to access the GSMA data.) The group should use the guiding questions to determine whether the country has sufficient existing technical infrastructure, patient data protections, and human resources to launch telemedicine services. Consider both these measures and planned expansions of existing services—that is, connectivity and smartphone penetration.

EXPRESS INTEREST AND COMMIT TO DEDICATING HUMAN RESOURCES TO FURTHER EXPLORE TELEMEDICINE OR HEALTH HOTLINE SERVICES

Once the government has confirmed the previous requirements, it should develop a formal commitment to establishing the service. This original expression of interest should be in writing, so it can be shared with different government ministries and relevant stakeholders to secure the human and financial resources needed to further explore development of the service.

ANNEX 2A. MINIMUM POLITICAL AND POLICY REQUIREMENTS TOOL

Purpose: The Minimum Political and Policy Requirements Tool helps governments assess the level of political stability, and of alignment of the solution with government policy and priorities, so they can decide whether to move forward with planning.

Timing: The ministry of health should use this tool before moving forward with planning for telemedicine or health hotline services in the country.

Instructions: The government should ask these questions at a high-level convening, such as a standard senior management meeting at the ministry of health. If the answer is no for stability, pursuing the services at this time would likely not be a good use of resources. The government can continue to address the political alignment, so a no might just signal the need for more groundwork. The political alignment will also help the government think through solution targeting—that is, the audience for the telemedicine or health hotline service and the health topics.

CATEGORY	QUESTION	REASON FOR QUESTION	ANSWER
Stability	Does the government currently have basic-level political stability (that is, is it stable and functioning to meet basic needs, or is there ongoing conflict)?	Needed to ensure decision-making and leadership for establishment of the service	
	Does the government anticipate a basic level of stability for at least two years (that is, are there upcoming elections or anticipated political changes that would affect solution champions)?	Needed to ensure continuity in solution leadership when implementing and embedding the services into the health system	
Political alignment	Does the proposed solution align with government policy? What types of services are allowed? Will the government approve a telemedicine service designed to diagnose and treat?	Needed to ensure solution is allowed at the most basic level before it can be included in strategies and budgets and have government champions	
	Do avenues exist for ensuring that prioritized activities, such as telemedicine or health hotline services, can be financed through the government for the long term?	Needed to ensure solution inclusion in budgets	
	Does the government have at least one focal high-level champion who will advocate for the solution to move forward?	Needed to ensure drive from the government	
	Does the proposed solution align with government priorities (investment and target geographies and beneficiaries)?	Needed to ensure solution inclusion in strategies and budgets, as well as to build government champions (Note: If the target geographies and beneficiaries the service will serve are already identified as priority areas and groups, it will be easier to make the case for the services.)	

ANNEX 2B. MINIMUM TECHNICAL CONSIDERATIONS CHECKLIST

Purpose: The Minimum Technical Considerations Checklist helps governments to review the existing technical capabilities and readiness of the health care system to adopt telemedicine or health hotlines. Although we do not define set targets for readiness, measuring and understanding where a country falls in the following measures of readiness will help to guide conversations on whether it is worth the investment at this time and what needs to happen to make sure the implementation of a telemedicine or health hotline program can be successful.

Timing: The ministry of health should use this tool before moving forward with planning for telemedicine or health hotline services in the country and after it has determined that it has the bare minimum political stability needed to move forward.

Instructions: The ministry of health, in consultation with the ministry of communication, should review the considerations at an existing forum. The person leading the discussion should bring any prior data to the meetings. Data may come from GSMA Intelligence (https://data.gsmaintelligence.com/signin? returnPath=%2Fdata%2Fcustom-metrics-search) or be documented in needs assessments or other internally generated reports. The group should use the guiding questions to determine whether the country has sufficient existing technical infrastructure, patient data protections, and human resources to launch telemedicine services. Consider both these measures and planned expansions of existing services—that is, connectivity and smartphone penetration.

TECHNICAL AND RESOURCES CONSIDERATIONS	POTENTIAL MEASURE
Internet connectivity	Number of internet contracts or internet service providers
Electrical availability and reliability	Percentage of population with access to electricity (https://data.worldbank.org/indicator/EG.ELC.ACCS.ZS)
Cell phone penetration	Percentage of population with access to basic mobile phone contracts
Smartphone penetration	Percentage of population with smartphone contracts
Availability of health care providers	Number of doctors, nurses and midwives, and clinical officers per capita
Existing data privacy and data protection processes in place	Validate with basic yes or no documentation
Availability of data storage/data center services (for countries requiring in-country data storage)	Number of data centers for data storage

Guiding questions based on data:

- Can the target population access the service that will be provided?

- What communication channels would be most successful given the existing infrastructure—that is, basic phone or audio via call center, interactive voice response messages, Unstructured Supplementary Service Data or Short Message Service, chatbots requiring smartphone, or video?

- Do you have sufficient staff to support the new technology—that is, call center staff, nurses, doctors, and so on?

- Are data protections sufficient and in line with global standards on patient data protection?

NOTES

1. Hussain (2014) defines political instability as "the propensity of a government collapse either because of conflicts or rampant competition between various political parties." According to a PESTEL analysis, political factors relevant to this toolkit include government policy and political stability or instability (see Professional Academy, no date).
2. See the GSMA *State of Mobile Internet Connectivity 2020* report (https://www.gsma.com /r/wp-content/uploads/2020/09/GSMA-State-of-Mobile-Internet-Connectivity-Report -2020.pdf) for information on the specific country context (Bahia and Delaporte 2020).

REFERENCES

Bahia, K., and A. Delaporte. 2020. *The State of Mobile Internet Connectivity 2020*. GSMA, London. https://www.gsma.com/r/wp-content/uploads/2020/09/GSMA-State-of -Mobile-Internet-Connectivity-Report-2020.pdf.

Handforth, C., and M. Wilson. 2019. *Digital Identity Country Report: Malawi*. GSMA, London. https://www.gsma.com/mobilefordevelopment/wp-content/uploads/2019/02/Digital -Identity-Country-Report.pdf.

Hussain, Z. 2014. "Can Political Stability Hurt Economic Growth?" *World Bank Blogs*, June 1, 2014. https://blogs.worldbank.org/endpovertyinsouthasia/can-political-stability-hurt -economic-growth.

Professional Academy. No date. "Marketing Theories—PESTEL Analysis." *Marketing Theories* (blog). https://www.professionalacademy.com/blogs-and-advice/marketing-theories ---pestel-analysis.

Scope and Design the Solution

During Phase 1, governments will scope and design the basic functional requirements of the solution. To do so, the government should identify a small planning task force, led by a focal point and dedicated to exploring the feasibility of the solution.

Chapter 3 helps governments understand the stakeholders needed for scoping and designing a solution. Chapter 4 helps governments understand how to establish the target audience, health topics, and potential uptake of the service; how to conduct a landscape analysis to determine available in-country resources; and, finally, how to use that preliminary information to develop a basic functional solution design.

Establish a Focal Point and Planning Task Force, and Understand the Champions Required for a Solution with Sustainable Impact at Scale

Chapter 3 helps the government appoint a focal point and form a planning task force. It also helps the government understand the key stakeholders needed to plan, implement, and sustain the solution. It presents two tools and a set of tips:

- *Terms of Reference for the Telemedicine or Health Hotline Planning Task Force (annex 3A)*
- *Telemedicine or Health Hotline Stakeholder Matrix (annex 3B)*
- *Tips for Coordinating across Departments, Ministries, and Partners (annex 3C)*

ESTABLISH A FOCAL POINT AND PLANNING TASK FORCE

The process of scoping and designing the solution can take time and therefore requires a planning task force and a focal point to lead it.[1] The purpose of the planning task force, which should be created by the ministry of health, is to scope and design the solution, and to develop a preliminary one-year road map and five-year strategy. Although the steering committee (formed in Phase 2), which acts as the decision-making body, will later review and approve the road map and strategy, the planning task force will continue to follow up on actions based on steering committee decisions. The planning task force should include representatives from different departments within the ministry of health, representatives from the relevant health regulatory bodies, a representative from the leading mobile network operators (MNOs), and service providers[2] and potential technical assistants. The ideal focal point for this task force would be someone from the ministry of health department that has shown interest in exploring potential services (typically, the clinical services or preventive care or health promotion department). The focal point selected should understand the dynamics between partners within the government and between governments and external stakeholders. This person should also have the power and ability to drive both informal and formal information gathering sessions with high-level officials. See the detailed Terms of Reference for the Telemedicine or Health Hotline Planning Task Force in annex 3A.

UNDERSTAND WHAT DEPARTMENTS, PARTNERS, AND OTHERS MAY BE NEEDED FOR INITIAL ESTABLISHMENT AND ONGOING SUSTAINABILITY

Regardless of solution design, ensuring solution sustainability requires several stakeholders. Critical stakeholders include various government ministries and departments as well as external stakeholders, such as MNOs, potential technical partners, and private sector service providers. The Telemedicine or Health Hotline Stakeholder Matrix in annex 3B helps governments understand which stakeholders are needed during the solution design, implementation, and scale phases. It also indicates if the stakeholder is required or optional, depending on the proposed solution design. This matrix can be used for planning strategic sessions, working groups, and steering committees. See the Tips for Coordinating across Departments, Ministries, and Partners in annex 3C for additional ways of working to create sustainable solution impact at scale.

Governments, through the focal point and planning task force, often need to have individual meetings to gather ideas before holding decision-making forums. Additionally, larger cross-sectoral meetings will be necessary for input and validation, as well as periodic meetings once the telemedicine or health hotline service is established and operating. Figure 3.1 lists the coordination types necessary for each step within each phase. Each government has different structures and may choose what works best, and it can determine how it can use existing government meetings to monitor implementation and scale-up.

FIGURE 3.1

Stakeholder coordination by phase and key milestones

Phases 0–1
- Assess basic requirements and express interest in writing to dedicate time and resources.
- Appoint individual focal point and form planning task force.
- Gather interest from each relevant department individually, and get input on prescoping, uptake assessment, and landscape analysis.
- Planning task force proposes initial functional solution design.

Phase 2
- Form steering committee and hold high-level functional design validation meeting.
- Planning task force develops draft five-year strategy.
- Planning task force forms partner selection committee to put out request for proposal to identify technology partners and get proposed budget amounts.
- Planning task force develops one-year road map to cost solution based on high-level design and potential partners to cost solution.
- Conduct five-year strategy, road map, and budget validation stakeholder meeting.

Phase 3
- Highest-level government official sends official letter to donors, partners, and ministry of finance expressing interest, budget, and need for funding.
- All relevant stakeholders solicit for funding.
- Focal department establishes memorandum of understanding with mobile network operators.

Phase 4
- For ongoing governance, continue to use steering committee or embed in existing coordination technical working groups or other subcommittees.
- Include services in any strategic plans and budget planning and validation processes.

Source: Original figure developed for this publication.

ANNEX 3A. TERMS OF REFERENCE FOR THE TELEMEDICINE OR HEALTH HOTLINE PLANNING TASK FORCE

Purpose: The purpose of the Terms of Reference for the Telemedicine or Health Hotline Planning Task Force is to help governments understand the purpose, roles, and membership of the planning task force that will scope and design the telemedicine or health hotline services, and to help the government and stakeholders design a five-year strategy and develop a one-year road map. This group needs to be dynamic and understand the roles for planning to move forward.

Timing: After determining that it meets the basic political and technical requirements, and once the ministry of health has identified the focal point in the department leading telemedicine or health hotline exploration, the government should form this task force at the very beginning of Phase 1.

Instructions: The focal point in the ministry of health, with authority from high-level officials in the ministry should reach out to the needed members included in the membership section, review the terms of reference, and begin supporting the government's planning for the services in the country. The focal point should fill the items in red with the relevant country context and make adjustments as needed.

INSERT COUNTRY X GOVERNMENT LOGO

TERMS OF REFERENCE FOR THE TELEMEDICINE OR HEALTH HOTLINE PLANNING TASK FORCE

Purpose

The purpose of the planning task force is to scope and design the [select: telemedicine, health hotline, or both telemedicine and health hotline] services, and to help the government and stakeholders develop a five-year strategy and one-year road map for review and validation by the decision-making [select: telemedicine, health hotline, or both telemedicine and health hotline] steering committee.

The [insert the lead department at the ministry of health for the services] leads this multisector small task force.

Specific responsibilities by relevant phases

Phase 0: Assess basic requirements and express interest
Phase 1: Scope and design solution
Phase 2: Develop strategy, implementation road map, and budget
Phase 3: Secure funding

Phases 0–2

- Attend all called meetings (Note: Meetings in Phases 0–2 may not occur at specific intervals but be called individually). Switching out members at regular meetings leads to delays and confusion.

- Develop, conduct, and analyze uptake and landscape analysis (or provide feedback to consultant) for validation by the [select: telemedicine, health hotline, or both telemedicine and health hotline] steering committee.
- Using input from key stakeholders and members of the [select: telemedicine, health hotline, or both telemedicine and health hotline] steering committee, develop high-level scope and solution design and solution description for [select: national telemedicine or hotline] services for validation by the [select: telemedicine, health hotline, or both telemedicine and health hotline] steering committee.
- Help the steering committee develop a five-year strategy, including vision for implementation and ongoing sustainability and establishing key performance indicators, and develop one-year road map for validation by the [select: telemedicine, health hotline, or both telemedicine and health hotline] steering committee.
- Help establish a subcommittee for partner selection to develop specific requests for proposals, review proposals, and select service providers (if applicable).
- Cost five-year strategy and one-year road map for validation by the [select: telemedicine, health hotline, or both telemedicine and health hotline] steering committee.
- Discuss options for, advocate for, and develop a plan for funding for [select: national telemedicine or hotline] services from respective government entities for validation by the [select: telemedicine, health hotline, or both telemedicine and health hotline] steering committee.
- Draft plan for any needed policy changes for validation by the [select: telemedicine, health hotline, or both telemedicine and health hotline] steering committee.
- Draft advertising and demand generation plan for the services for validation by the [select: telemedicine, health hotline, or both telemedicine and health hotline] steering committee.

Phase 3

- Develop proposals based on the validated scope, plans, and budgets.
- Brainstorm options for, advocate for, and develop a plan and assign roles for securing an agreement with MNOs to provide short codes and zero-rate incoming calls (at minimum) and to advertise the service via free blasts (when allowable by the communications regulators in the specified country).

Phase 4

Not applicable

General

Provide updates to [select: national telemedicine or hotline] steering committee.

Timing

The multisector [select: national telemedicine or hotline] planning task force will meet as needed to complete Phases 0–3, which will likely take a concentrated amount of work for a 3–6 month period.

Membership

The planning task force membership shall include the following (Department membership depends on the scope of the [select: national telemedicine or hotline] services provided; see the stakeholder matrix). Note that stakeholders listed are based on the official titles of the Malawi stakeholders involved in the Chipatala Cha Pa Foni, or Health Center by Phone, solution. Each government has different titles and structures and will need to adapt the titles as relevant.

- Ministry of Health
  - Directorate of Clinical Services (required) and whatever department or directorate is chosen to steward the services
  - Directorate of Preventive Health Services—Health Education Services (required)
  - Department of Planning and Policy Development (required)
  - Department of Information and Communication Technology (if one exists within the Ministry of Health and one for the government as a whole, the ministry department would be more relevant) (required)
  - Department of Administration and Finance (in the Ministry of Health) (required)
  - Medical specialty departments (dermatology, mental health, and so on) (required for telemedicine; optional for health hotline)
- Health regulatory bodies (Medical or Nurses Council)
- Representative from major MNOs that would be linked to the services
- Service providers, once selected

ANNEX 3B. TELEMEDICINE OR HEALTH HOTLINE STAKEHOLDER MATRIX

Purpose: The Telemedicine or Health Hotline Stakeholder Matrix helps governments understand who specifically is needed during solution design, implementation, scale, and sustainability phases. It also indicates if the stakeholder is required or optional with a given solution design.

Timing: The matrix is worth reviewing when beginning to plan; at minimum, the ministry of health department that is leading the planning and has appointed the focal point should review it before beginning any scoping activities.

Instructions: The focal point, planning committee, and director of the department leading the services in the long term should use this matrix for planning strategic sessions, working groups, steering committees, and so on.

Please note, stakeholders listed in the matrix are based on the official titles of the Malawi stakeholders involved in the Chipatala Cha Pa Foni, or Health Center by Phone, solution. Each government has different titles and structures, and governments will need to adapt the titles as relevant.

TYPE OF ORGANIZATION AND TITLE OF DEPARTMENT/ DIVISION/ORGANIZATION	GENERAL ROLE OF DEPARTMENT/DIVISION/ ORGANIZATION	REASON NEEDED FOR TELEMEDICINE OR HEALTH HOTLINE	WHO IS NEEDED AT WHICH STAGE OF THE PROCESS? PHASE 0: ASSESS BASIC REQUIREMENTS AND EXPRESS INTEREST PHASE 1: SCOPE AND DESIGN SOLUTION PHASE 2: DEVELOP STRATEGY, IMPLEMENTATION ROAD MAP, AND BUDGET PHASE 3: SECURE FUNDING FOR START-UP PERIOD PHASE 4: ESTABLISH, IMPLEMENT, SCALE, AND SUSTAIN SOLUTION	REQUIRED OR OPTIONAL
Ministry of Health (MOH): Minister of Health or Secretary for Health	Provide the overall strategic direction for the MOH	• Ultimate decision-maker on whether health hotlines or telemedicine services could and should be offered as part of the overall health system • Sign official strategic plans and budgets	Minister of Health and Secretary for Health: • *Phase 0:* Need to be informed and generally agree with exploring services. • *Phase 1:* Not needed in initial discussions but should sign off on final scope to ensure alignment with strategic vision and country-specific regulations. • *Phase 2:* Five-year strategic planning: Minister of Health, Secretary for Health, or both should sign off on the strategic plan but are not needed in the planning. They should provide guidance for which department would be responsible for stewarding the service. Not needed for one-year road map/ establishment. • *Phase 3:* Officially issue document request to Ministry of Finance to get the services added to budgets. Midlevel managers generally write the letter of request, but the minister and secretary sign it. • *Phase 4:* Not needed for establishment and implementation. Scale (ongoing sustainability management): Need to sign off on future strategic plans and budgets in accordance with the five-year strategy.	Required
MOH: Directorate of Clinical Services	Provides strategic direction and oversight of all clinical and emergency services	At a minimum for both: • Ensures the telemedicine or health hotline connects to the existing clinical and emergency services when a caller presents with danger signs Telemedicine: • Lead steward would likely fall under this department Hotline: • Would depend on the country. In Malawi, Clinical Services is responsible for Health Center by Phone; in Mozambique, the hotline sits in the Health Promotion Department	Director of Clinical Services needed for sign-off in Phases 0, 1, and 2 (five-year strategic plan). Role in Phases 3 or 4 may vary depending on services offered and where the services sit. For example, if telemedicine or if Clinical Services stewards the hotline, the director would be critical for any oversight and sign-off in Phases 3 and 4. Midlevel technocrat (deputy and below): May be aware of and drive each phase, but the strategic sign-offs must be at the highest level in the department. Phase 4 would predominantly fall at this level. Manager: If this directorate stewards the services, it will need a direct focal point to oversee Phase 4.	Required for both telemedicine and health hotlines, but level of involvement depends on whether one or both are being implemented

continued

TYPE OF ORGANIZATION AND TITLE OF DEPARTMENT/ DIVISION/ORGANIZATION	GENERAL ROLE OF DEPARTMENT/DIVISION/ ORGANIZATION	REASON NEEDED FOR TELEMEDICINE OR HEALTH HOTLINE	WHO IS NEEDED AT WHICH STAGE OF THE PROCESS? PHASE 0: ASSESS BASIC REQUIREMENTS AND EXPRESS INTEREST PHASE 1: SCOPE AND DESIGN SOLUTION PHASE 2: DEVELOP STRATEGY, IMPLEMENTATION ROAD MAP, AND BUDGET PHASE 3: SECURE FUNDING FOR START-UP PERIOD PHASE 4: ESTABLISH, IMPLEMENT, SCALE, AND SUSTAIN SOLUTION	REQUIRED OR OPTIONAL
MOH: Directorate of Preventive Health Services—Health Education Services	Provides communities with information on health services and campaigns and provides health prevention information	At a minimum for both: • Promotes the telemedicine and health hotline services through existing promotion channels, personnel, and collateral Health hotline: • In Mozambique, the Health Promotion Department (equivalent) stewards the hotline	Deputy Director of Preventive Health Services—Health Education Services needed for sign-off in Phases 0, 1, and 2 (five-year strategic plan). Role in Phases 3 or 4 varies depending on services offered and where the services sit. For example, for health hotlines, if this directorate stewards the hotline, it would be critical for any oversight and sign-off in Phases 3 and 4. Midlevel technocrat manager (deputy and below): May be aware of and drive each phase, but the strategic sign-offs must be at the highest level in the department. Needed for Phase 2 planning for both five-year strategy and one-year road map. Phase 4 would predominantly fall at this level. Manager: If this directorate stewards the services, it will need a direct focal point to oversee Phase 4.	Required
MOH: Directorate of Preventive Health Services—Community Health Department	Provides direct services in the community and provides communities with health information	At a minimum for both: • Ensures community health workers are aware of the telemedicine or health hotline services and promote them to communities (and among each other, if provided in the service design) Health hotline: • May steward hotline, and operators could be from the community health workers cadre	Deputy Director of Community Health Services needed for sign-off in Phases 0, 1, and 2 (five-year strategic plan). Role in Phases 3 or 4 varies depending on services offered and where the services sit. For example, if telemedicine or if community health stewards the hotline, they would be critical for any oversight and sign-off in Phases 3 and 4. Midlevel technocrat (deputy and below): May be aware of and drive each phase, but the strategic sign-offs must be at the highest level in the department. Phase 4 would predominantly fall at this level.	Required
MOH: Department of Planning and Policy Development—Central Monitoring and Evaluation Division	Provides oversight of MOH activities, tracks key performance indicators, and ensures integration of data	• Ensures that data captured in the telemedicine or health hotline service meet the needs of the government • Establishes key performance indicators • Ensures dashboards and data from the services are shared and available across departments • Develops (or codevelops with the Digital Health Division) data-sharing agreement	Deputy Director of Monitoring and Evaluation needed for sign-off on Phases 0, 1, and 2 (five-year strategic plan). Mid- or lower-level technocrat (deputy and below): Phase 4 would predominantly fall at this level. Officer level would be responsible for analysis of data from the services.	Required (if this division exists)

continued

TYPE OF ORGANIZATION AND TITLE OF DEPARTMENT/ DIVISION/ORGANIZATION	GENERAL ROLE OF DEPARTMENT/DIVISION/ ORGANIZATION	REASON NEEDED FOR TELEMEDICINE OR HEALTH HOTLINE	WHO IS NEEDED AT WHICH STAGE OF THE PROCESS? PHASE 0: ASSESS BASIC REQUIREMENTS AND EXPRESS INTEREST; PHASE 1: SCOPE AND DESIGN SOLUTION; PHASE 2: DEVELOP STRATEGY, IMPLEMENTATION ROAD MAP, AND BUDGET; PHASE 3: SECURE FUNDING FOR START-UP PERIOD; PHASE 4: ESTABLISH, IMPLEMENT, SCALE, AND SUSTAIN SOLUTION	REQUIRED OR OPTIONAL
MOH: Department of Planning and Policy Development—Quality Management Division	Provides oversight of quality of MOH services	• Develops quality assurance requirements and policies for telemedicine or health hotline services • Conducts spot checks on quality assurance assessments	Deputy Director of Quality Management needed for sign-off in Phases 0, 1, and 2 (five-year strategic plan). Mid- or lower-level technocrat (deputy and below): Phase 4 would predominantly fall at this level. Officer level would be responsible for conducting spot checks on the quarterly quality assurance assessments done by the supervisors of the telemedicine or hotline services.	Required (if this division exists)
MOH: Department of Planning and Policy Development—Digital Health Division (in some countries sits outside of the MOH and is an e-strategy division in the government)	Develops the e-strategy; ensures partners align with registration, reporting, and integration of digital data and systems; and may be responsible for the internet and server infrastructure	• Develops requirements for and provides oversight of how the telemedicine or health hotline should work with other systems (and defines which are relevant) and follow the overall e-strategy (if applicable) requirements • Approves data-sharing agreements	Deputy Director of Digital Health needed for sign-off in Phases 0, 1, and 2 (five-year strategic plan). Mid- or lower-level technocrat (deputy and below): Phase 4 would predominantly fall at this level. Officer: Responsible for enforcing and helping with interoperability and data-sharing agreements between the MOH, communications, mobile network operators, and relevant stakeholders (if components are outsourced) in Phase 4.	Required (if this division exists)
MOH: Department of Information and Communication Technology (if one exists within the MOH and another for the government as a whole, the one in MOH would be more relevant)	Provides direct information and communication, repairs technology, manages MOH software systems, and so on	• Provides basic management of the telemedicine or health hotline hardware and software • May be responsible for upgrading system, unless all information and communication technology services are outsourced to service providers	Director of Information and Communication Technology needed for sign-off on Phases 0, 1, and 2 (five-year strategic plan); would also need to appoint a lower-level officer for Phase 4 to ensure ongoing maintenance and upgrades if the services are offered in-house. Lower-level technocrat: Phase 4 would predominantly fall at this level. Officer level would be responsible for ongoing maintenance or alerting outsourced service providers of issues if the hotline is physically located at the MOH but other providers maintain the software and hardware.	Required (if this division exists)
MOH: Department of Planning and Policy Development	Oversees the development of strategic plans and budgets across the ministry	• Validates memorandums of understandings with partners and service providers • Ensures telemedicine or health hotline services are embedded in strategic plans and budgets	Director needed for sign-off on Phases 0, 1, and 2 (five-year strategic plan); also needed for Phase 4 during scaling and sustainability to ensure the solution continues to be embedded in the strategic plans and budgets.	Required (if this division exists)

continued

TYPE OF ORGANIZATION AND TITLE OF DEPARTMENT/ DIVISION/ORGANIZATION	GENERAL ROLE OF DEPARTMENT/DIVISION/ ORGANIZATION	REASON NEEDED FOR TELEMEDICINE OR HEALTH HOTLINE	WHO IS NEEDED AT WHICH STAGE OF THE PROCESS? PHASE 0: ASSESS BASIC REQUIREMENTS AND EXPRESS INTEREST PHASE 1: SCOPE AND DESIGN SOLUTION PHASE 2: DEVELOP STRATEGY, IMPLEMENTATION ROAD MAP, AND BUDGET PHASE 3: SECURE FUNDING FOR START-UP PERIOD PHASE 4: ESTABLISH, IMPLEMENT, SCALE, AND SUSTAIN SOLUTION	REQUIRED OR OPTIONAL
MOH: Department of Administration and Finance (in the MOH)	Approves, monitors, and releases MOH funding received from the Ministry of Finance to the respective MOH departments	• Releases funding to the department stewarding the telemedicine or health hotline services, whether in-house or outsourced	Director of Administration and Finance needed for sign-off in Phases 0, 1, and 2 (five-year strategic plan). Midlevel manager needed to release funding in Phases 3 and 4 for payment, either directly to the MOH department or directly to the service provider for outsourced services.	Required
MOH: Department of Human Resources	Develops the human resource establishment list and oversees hiring in the MOH	Role depends on whether services are fully or partially outsourced or in-house. If in-house: • Adds telemedicine or hotline workers to human resources establishment • Recruits telemedicine or human resources workers	Director of Human Resources needed for sign-off in Phases 0, 1, and 2 (five-year strategic plan) only if in-house. Deputy or next level: If in-house, needed in Phase 4 for ongoing hiring and ensuring personnel continue to be included in the official establishment.	Required if in-house; may be optional if outsourced, depending on mandate of the division
MOH: Departments related to specific health topics (maternal, newborn, and child health; sexual and reproductive services; Expanded Programme on Immunization; nutrition; noncommunicable diseases; tuberculosis; malaria; and so on)	Provide strategic direction, policies, guidelines, and oversight for MOH activities for their specific health focus area	May be needed if telemedicine or health hotline services on all health topics are needed For each department in design scope (whether in-house or outsourced): • Provide initial validation of the health content, training needs, and so on • Make periodic upgrades to the content, frequently asked questions, and training based on changes in MOH official policy and content to delete outdated information	If the telemedicine or health hotline services solution design includes all health topics, each director is needed for sign-off in Phases 0, 1, and 2 (five-year strategic plan); for helping pool funding or advocate for funding in Phase 3; and for sign-off on including topics in the overall strategic plans for sustainability in the scaling section of Phase 4. Midlevel technocrat (deputy and below): If all health topics, each technocrat assigned from all the departments would need to do initial validation of the health content, training needs, and so on; would also be responsible for periodic upgrades to the content, frequently asked questions, and training based on changes in MOH official policy and content to ensure deletion of outdated information. Phase 4 would predominantly fall at this level. Needed whether or not the services are outsourced because of the importance of providing the most accurate information, advice, and so on.	All required if the services are for all health topics The government may choose to have telemedicine or health hotline focus on just one of these areas; if so, that department would be the steward of the service and the others would not be needed

continued

TYPE OF ORGANIZATION AND TITLE OF DEPARTMENT/DIVISION/ORGANIZATION	GENERAL ROLE OF DEPARTMENT/DIVISION/ORGANIZATION	REASON NEEDED FOR TELEMEDICINE OR HEALTH HOTLINE	WHO IS NEEDED AT WHICH STAGE OF THE PROCESS? PHASE 0: ASSESS BASIC REQUIREMENTS AND EXPRESS INTEREST / PHASE 1: SCOPE AND DESIGN SOLUTION / PHASE 2: DEVELOP STRATEGY, IMPLEMENTATION ROAD MAP, AND BUDGET / PHASE 3: SECURE FUNDING FOR START-UP PERIOD / PHASE 4: ESTABLISH, IMPLEMENT, SCALE, AND SUSTAIN SOLUTION	REQUIRED OR OPTIONAL
MOH: Medical specialty departments (dermatology, mental health, and so on)	Provide medical specialty services to patients	• Provide telemedicine services to patients • Provide guidance to health care providers in remote areas (if in solution scope) • Not needed for a health hotline, except as a referral option (would provide the contacts to the hotline workers)	Directors of respective clinical services/medical specialty departments needed for sign-off in Phases 0, 1, and 2 (five-year strategic plan for telemedicine services); also need to help regulatory departments align on policy. Medical specialists: If in-house, needed in Phase 4 for ongoing telemedicine services. If outsourced, the government may want some of its specialists to provide periodic quality assurance audits.	Required for telemedicine Optional or not required for health hotline
Health regulatory bodies: Medical or Nurses Council	Develop and enforce policies for the implementation of health-related services	• Help develop and enforce telemedicine policies (may be joint effort with the Ministry of Communication) • Determine needed policies for health hotlines	Director of the Medical or Nurses Council needed for sign-off on Phases 0, 1, and 2 (five-year strategic plan for telemedicine services); also needed to help develop regulatory policy and enforcement in Phase 4. Members of regulatory body: Needed for Phase 4 enforcement.	Required for telemedicine and hotlines that have clinical staff (nurses and above); may be optional for hotlines with lower-level cadres
Ministry of Communication: Communications regulatory body	Develops and enforces policies for the implementation of information systems, mobile network operators, and so on	• Helps establish communication regulations related to telemedicine or health hotlines • Brokers agreements with mobile network operators for reduced cost (for government) for telemedicine or health hotline services	Director may be needed for sign-off on any policies and plans in Phases 0, 1, and 2. Midlevel director needed for Phase 4 and needed to broker agreements with mobile network operators.	Required
Ministry of Justice: Secretary for Justice	Reviews memorandums of understanding and official strategic documents for legal ramifications	• Approves memorandums of understanding with mobile network operators and service providers of telemedicine or health hotline services • Approves official strategic documents for legal ramifications	Secretary for Justice needed for sign-off on any official memorandums of understanding, policies, and so on. For telemedicine or health hotlines, sign-off may come at Phase 2, Phase 2–3 (for agreements with mobile network operators), or Phase 4.	Required
Ministry of Finance: Minister of Finance or Secretary to the Treasury	Approves and releases funding for all government ministries	• Approves and releases funding for telemedicine or health hotline services	Minister of Finance: Phase 2 sign-off of five-year strategy and any agreements with service providers; Phase 3 approval and disbursement of any internal funding.	Required
Mobile network operators: All major mobile network operators in country	Provide telecommunication services throughout the country	• Provide short codes for government telemedicine or health hotline • Zero-rate or reduce call costs for government to allow for free calls for users nationwide, and advertise services through networks	Director: Needed in Phases 2, 3, and 4 for sign-off on any agreements with the government (preferably) or service providers. Midlevel manager: Needed to manage relationship and implementation in Phases 3 and 4.	Required

continued

TYPE OF ORGANIZATION AND TITLE OF DEPARTMENT/DIVISION/ORGANIZATION	GENERAL ROLE OF DEPARTMENT/DIVISION/ORGANIZATION	REASON NEEDED FOR TELEMEDICINE OR HEALTH HOTLINE	WHO IS NEEDED AT WHICH STAGE OF THE PROCESS? PHASE 0: ASSESS BASIC REQUIREMENTS AND EXPRESS INTEREST; PHASE 1: SCOPE AND DESIGN SOLUTION; PHASE 2: DEVELOP STRATEGY, IMPLEMENTATION ROAD MAP, AND BUDGET; PHASE 3: SECURE FUNDING FOR START-UP PERIOD; PHASE 4: ESTABLISH, IMPLEMENT, SCALE, AND SUSTAIN SOLUTION	REQUIRED OR OPTIONAL
Donors: Relevant multilateral, bilateral, or other donors	Provide direct funding to the government or other partners for general government-identified priorities for digital health or telemedicine or other related services	• Provide funding for the setup and initial implementation of the telemedicine or health hotline infrastructure or services until the government can partially or wholly sustain the service in its budgets	Midlevel managers needed for each phase (director needs to ultimately sign off on overall budget for Phase 3 and ongoing, for as long as projected in strategic plan for Phase 4).	Required unless the government can fully fund setup and ongoing implementation or outsourcing agreement
Service providers: Private telemedicine companies, private hotline companies, nongovernmental organizations, or other providers of technology and services needed for telemedicine or health hotlines (may include technical assistance)	Provide services for customer	• Operate and manage or establish telemedicine or hotline services • Maintain technology needed (hotline platforms, dashboards, interactive voice response, Short Message Service, WhatsApp, and so on)	Directors ultimately sign off on any agreements, but midlevel managers needed for ongoing arrangements and planning for each phase.	Required if any part of the setup and implementation is outsourced or provided by parties external to government
Other partners: Any relevant partners, such as nongovernmental organizations and academic institutions, that support or promote MOH services	Provide financial support, technical assistance, and direct implementation to MOH	At minimum for both: • Advertise the telemedicine or health hotline services through their networks and embed numbers on collateral • May support or implement setup and ongoing implementation until point of transition to the government or could provide planning technical assistance	Midlevel managers needed for Phases 1–2 if they are the partner the government asks for planning, technical assistance, or implementation. Directors needed for Phase 3 budget sign-off. Midlevel managers needed for Phase 4. Officers or hotline workers (level of cadre dependent on government requirements) needed for Phase 4 if not yet embedded in government establishment.	Optional depending on how the government approaches planning, setup, and implementation

ANNEX 3C. TIPS FOR COORDINATING ACROSS DEPARTMENTS, MINISTRIES, AND PARTNERS

Each phase involved in establishing a solution requires many stakeholders, departments, and ministries, and coordination across these stakeholders can be complex. Journey to Sustainability and Scale with Government (https://www .villagereach.org/wp-content/uploads/2022/10/Stakeholder-Alignment _Overview.pdf) offers a basic tool to help governments, donors, and partners work toward sustainability from the outset (VillageReach 2022). Additionally, coordination across stakeholders requires the following:

- Be open, honest, collaborative, and communicative throughout the process.
  - *Tip:* Assign a point person to inform relevant stakeholders of progress, send and coordinate invitations to meetings, and so on.
- Align on the ultimate goals and key milestones from the beginning.
  - *Tip:* See the overview in VillageReach's "Journey to Sustainability and Scale with Government" (https://www.villagereach.org/wp-content /uploads/2022/10/Stakeholder-Alignment_Overview.pdf) for an option of how to achieve this alignment (VillageReach 2022).
- Document in writing all important decisions—critical in government because of personnel changes.
  - *Tip:* The government should work with any external partners to develop a memorandum of understanding early in the process.
- Identify early the key personnel, key decision-makers, and critical ministry departments and regulatory bodies.
  - *Tip:* Clarify roles and responsibilities; such clarification might require a RACI matrix (https://thedigitalprojectmanager.com/projects/leadership -team-management/raci-chart-made-simple/)—"responsible" (doer), "accountable" (decision-maker), "consulted," and "informed."[3]
  - *Tip:* Have the right people at the table at the right time. (Note: For a decentralized government, stakeholders should include representatives from counties, provinces, and districts.)
- Use existing government meetings (monthly, quarterly, and so on) and decision-making structures.
  - *Tip:* Adjust coordination processes, frequency, and structures if they are not helping drive toward the solution's key milestones.

NOTES

1. The planning task force and focal point are not the only way to set up the services, but experience shows that it helps to have a designated person responsible and a team for support to move things forward. Without a designated team, government officials find it hard to dedicate the time to move things forward. The members can still continue with their other work, but they would be expected to report back to their supervisors on progress as well.
2. Involving call center and technical service providers before the contracting (Phase 4) needs to be done in a way that complies with procurement rules; however, mobile network operators can be engaged very early in the process for zero-rating calls, short codes, and so on, and a memorandum of understanding would be in place by Phase 3.

3. For an explanation and example of a RACI chart, see Haworth (no date) at https://thedigitalprojectmanager.com/projects/leadership-team-management/raci-chart-made-simple/.

REFERENCES

Haworth, S. No date. "How to Create a RACI Chart: What Project Managers Need to Know." Digital Project Manager. https://thedigitalprojectmanager.com/projects/leadership-team-management/raci-chart-made-simple/.

Village Reach. 2022. "The Journey to Sustainability and Scale with Government: Introduction to Stakeholder Alignment Workshop Approach and Materials." https://www.villagereach.org/wp-content/uploads/2022/10/Stakeholder-Alignment_Overview.pdf.

Establish Target Audience, Select Health Areas, Understand Potential Uptake, Conduct Landscape Analysis, and Develop Basic Solution Design

Chapter 4 helps governments understand stakeholder perspectives and make critical decisions on the target audience and health topics, understand potential uptake from both the community and health workers, understand what existing partners and technologies the government can leverage, develop a national plan for coordinating multiple telemedicine or health hotline services, and develop a basic functional design for the appropriate solution. This chapter presents the following tools:

- *Telemedicine or Health Hotline Predesign Scoping Tool (annex 4A)*
- *Telemedicine or Health Hotline Services Uptake Assessment Tool (annex 4B)*
- *Landscape Analysis Tool: Questionnaire and Analysis Reflection Guide for Government and Stakeholders (annex 4C)*
- *Telemedicine or Health Hotline Solution Design Decision-Making Tool (annex 4D)*

TARGETING: DEFINE HEALTH AREA GAPS

Telemedicine or health hotline services can cover many health topics and populations. To plan for telemedicine or health hotline services, the government must first define the scope of the solution it wants to establish. It can use the Telemedicine or Health Hotline Predesign Scoping Tool in annex 4A to help define this scope. The decision tree in figure 4.1 provides the logical framework for the tool and helps answer two critical questions:

FIGURE 4.1

Predesign scoping decision tree for telemedicine or health hotline services

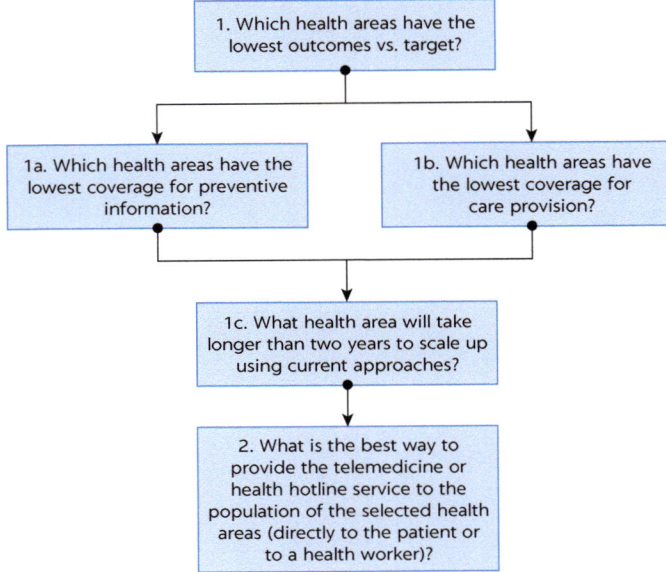

1. Which health areas have the lowest outcomes vs. target?

1a. Which health areas have the lowest coverage for preventive information?

1b. Which health areas have the lowest coverage for care provision?

1c. What health area will take longer than two years to scale up using current approaches?

2. What is the best way to provide the telemedicine or health hotline service to the population of the selected health areas (directly to the patient or to a health worker)?

1. What health areas (maternal, newborn, and child health; sexual and reproductive health; and others) should be prioritized given existing health outcomes and the national health strategy?

2. Which priority health areas have the lowest coverage (access) for preventive information? For care (diagnosis, treatment, prescription)? In terms of coverage, what are the priority health areas and health topics (for example, prenatal tips and reminders)? By health area, is preventative information or care provision the priority for the next five years?

3. With current health worker capacity plus planned hires over the next five years, are there any coverage gaps that could take more than two years to fill, even assuming funding is in place? The areas with a gap of two years or more should be your health hotline or telemedicine priorities.

4. What is the target audience for the health hotline or telemedicine service? Should it be provided directly to the patient or to a health worker?

Source: Original figure developed for this publication.

1. Which health areas should be covered (that is, which have the lowest health outcomes, lowest coverage, and longest time to fill coverage gaps)?
2. What is the best way to reach the population for the selected health areas (that is, directly to the patient or to a health worker)?

This tool is specifically for governments that have perceived health system gaps. Easy to use and requiring little in the way of time or resources, this tool helps governments fully document and understand their health system gaps. Understanding and documenting health system gaps will help governments understand their goals for implementing these services.

ASSESS THE STRUCTURAL AND CULTURAL FACTORS THAT MAY AFFECT SOLUTION SUCCESS

The uptake of telemedicine or health hotline services can be influenced by individual and structural factors, as well as by the characteristics of solution design (for example, perceived ease and benefits and cost of service). Conducting an uptake assessment will help the government understand what type of services target populations are likely to use.[1]

The Uptake Assessment Tool in annex 4B allows the government to make critical decisions about whether to implement the service, to determine what is required for acceptance, and to tailor the services to meet the needs of the target population. For example, if the ministry of health decides to make the solution available to all populations, the information gathered from the assessment can help the government promote and advocate for the services to different audiences. If the focal point or the other members of the planning task force are not available to conduct the assessment, the government should find a partner to conduct a thorough uptake analysis. (Note: If an analysis of this type has already been conducted, the government can leverage those results.) After the analysis has been conducted, its results should be presented to any members of the small planning task force who were not involved in the assessment so that they can help guide solution development.

This assessment should take one or two people about one to two weeks to perform. It does not require a statistically significant sample size; a purposive sample of 5–10 community members per comparison group (such as rural versus urban or northern region of the country versus southern region of the country) and 2–3 health workers per comparison group would be acceptable. The analysis team should conduct preliminary analysis of the assessment results to decide if this sample size is sufficient to understand the context or if additional respondents are needed. To leverage existing structures and reduce costs, governments could use community health workers or existing community health promotion channels to get interviewees. Additionally, governments may find useful the Pan American Health Organization's "COVID-19 and Telemedicine: Tool for Assessing the Maturity Level of Health Institutions to Implement Telemedicine Services" (https://www3.paho.org/ish/images/toolkit/COVID-19 -Telemedicine_RATool-en.pdf?ua=1) (PAHO and IDB 2020), which helps health institutions determine their readiness to provide telemedicine services. The tool is broken into six categories: organizational readiness, processes, digital environment, human resources, regulatory issues, and expertise.

ASSESS AVAILABLE IN-COUNTRY RESOURCES: CONDUCTING A LANDSCAPE ANALYSIS

Leveraging existing resources within a country is an important step before solution design. This section helps the government identify available resources that can support development and implementation. Because many types of digital health services and technologies exist, however, governments should focus on existing telemedicine or health hotline services and additional technologies that could enhance them (for example, interactive voice response, Short Message Service, Unstructured Supplementary Service Data, and WhatsApp).[2] The Landscape Analysis Tool in annex 4C aims to create an inventory of existing services to help governments make decisions on the following:

- What partners exist to help build out the services?
- What infrastructure or technologies already exist that can be used to reduce costs, prevent overlap, and promote integration and interoperability?
- What remaining gaps has the government, or other stakeholders, identified?

The landscape analysis should take one or two people about one to two weeks to perform using the Landscape Analysis Tool, depending on the availability of interviewees. The tool includes questions that will allow interviewees to point the interviewer to other services and organizations, creating a chain referral sampling and identifying potential partners to contact. For example, if a health hotline exists that includes the government's targeted health topics, the government could work with that partner to scale the hotline nationwide, or it could contract that partner to help the government establish its own in-house service.

As with the stakeholder alignment, it is critical to get all stakeholders convening (physically or virtually) regularly to avoid overlap, duplication of resources, and confusion. Using the landscape analysis, a focal point in the government can convene all service providers that deliver telemedicine or health hotline services or that provide supporting technology. If multiple services exist within the country, the government might consider forming a subcommittee to move forward with a national plan for aligning these services.

DESIGN A HIGH-LEVEL SOLUTION

The appointed planning task force should move forward on a basic functional solution design. The Telemedicine or Health Hotline Solution Design Decision-Making Tool in annex 4D helps develop the solution. It includes *functional design*, determining the functional scope (health area and audience), and *technical design*, which identifies the different technologies the solution will use (for example, hotline software with interactive voice response, WhatsApp, and so on). After the planning task force has results from this tool, the government will be ready to move into Phase 3, in which the steering committee will validate the initial design.

ANNEX 4A. TELEMEDICINE OR HEALTH HOTLINE PREDESIGN SCOPING TOOL

Purpose: The Predesign Scoping Tool helps governments reflect on the health areas with the greatest needs in the existing health system, determine which areas would take longer than two years to achieve targets using current approaches, and determine what audience (health care worker or direct to client) the solution would need to target to fill existing gaps.

Timing: This assessment should be completed after the government has conducted a brief gap analysis, about the same time it conducts the Uptake Assessment (see annex 4B), because both would help answer basic targeting questions for solution design of the telemedicine or health hotline services.

Instructions: This tool is targeted at government officials and can be conducted during a cross-departmental meeting with department heads at the ministry of health (such as a senior management meeting). A focal point leading the drive for the services from the planning task force should (1) conduct basic literature research of existing data on health care gaps and (2) lead a facilitated discussion with the senior management team at the ministry of health. Drawing the decisions on a white- or chalkboard may help visualize decisions.

Governments should adapt this tool to the context and include translation, as needed.

Script: *Thank you for allowing the time to be here with the senior management team today. I am [name of government focal point] from the [name of department at the ministry of health], and I am a member of the government planning task force exploring the possibility of adding telemedicine or health hotline services to our health system offerings. Before this discussion, key personnel at the ministry reviewed the basic political and technical requirements needed for telemedicine or health hotline services and have determined that [name of country] meets those basic requirements for [select: telemedicine, health hotline, or telemedicine and health hotlines]. [Show any data or results from the basic requirements reviews.]*

Note: If the country does not meet the bare minimum technical requirements for telemedicine at this time, the facilitator may want to focus from here on the "a" questions in question 2 and onward, which relate to health hotlines.

Today we will discuss what the health area priorities are based on the current situation in the country. This discussion will help us determine which areas to prioritize when developing a health hotline.

#	Question	Facilitator to reference existing data from departmental strategic plans, health surveys, gap analyses, and so on	Response	Note to facilitator
1	Which health areas (maternal, newborn, and child health; sexual and reproductive health; HIV; noncommunicable diseases; mental health; and so on) have the lowest outcomes relative to the target?			Have the data available, but also open the question to the government, which will have knowledge of additional resources. Try to get participants to list the health areas in order of greatest to least need.

continued

#	Question	Facilitator to reference existing data from departmental strategic plans, health surveys, gap analyses, and so on	Response	Note to facilitator
2a	Based on the results from question 1, which of these health areas have the lowest coverage for preventive information (access)?			2a results relate to health hotlines and messaging services.
2b	Based on the results from question 1, which of these health areas have the lowest coverage for care provision (diagnosis, treatment, and prescription)?			2b results relate to telemedicine services.
2c	By health areas identified in 1, 2a, and 2b, is prevention or care a priority for the next five years?			These results will help the government prioritize what would make more sense to focus on. If prevention comes out strongly, a hotline would be ideally suited; if care does, telemedicine could help with the gap. If both, the government may choose a phased approach to build out both.
3a	Based on results from 2a, which of the health areas will not be able to scale up preventive measures to meet targets within a two-year period using the existing planned interventions?			3a results relate to health hotlines and messaging services. Items that cannot reach their targets or do not have avenues of meeting the target would be a priority area for the hotline services.
3b	Based on results from 2b, which of the health areas will not be able to scale up care measures to meet targets within a two-year period using the existing planned interventions (that is, will human resource coverage gaps persist for two or more years)? Which cadres have the largest gaps that will take the longest to fill? Are these areas that can be handled by telemedicine?			3b results relate to telemedicine services. Items that cannot reach their targets or do not have avenues of meeting the target would be a priority area for telemedicine. Note which cadres need to be prioritized and if they can or cannot be filled by telemedicine. For example, telemedicine could not fill gaps in emergency services, surgery, and so on.

continued

#	Question	Facilitator to reference existing data from departmental strategic plans, health surveys, gap analyses, and so on	Response	Note to facilitator
3c	Based on the answers from 3b, can some cadres be given additional skills if provided with adequate supervision (that is, could access to supervisor-level personnel via telemedicine expand the ability to perform those services at a lower level)?			Telemedicine could be used for health workers or direct to consumers. The answers to 3c will help with question 5.
4	SKIP #4 (Structural and cultural factors)			Explain that the next logical question concerns structural and cultural factors, and explain where the team is in the process of the structural and cultural assessment. If not yet completed, explain what will be done; if completed, show the results and discuss.
5	Based on all the previous answers, what is the target audience for the service (health workers or direct to client)?			Based on all the evidence and needs, the government can decide where to focus efforts (on the health worker or direct to client). It can do both in the long term but should prioritize which should come first.
	Based on all the feedback, do we have alignment on the following? 1. The order of priority health areas is [list in order]. 2. The ministry of health would like to focus on a service [select: for health workers or direct to consumer]. 3. The ministry of health would like to [select: focus on a health hotline, focus on telemedicine, or set up a health hotline first and then expand to telemedicine].			Gaining consensus is critical so that the small task force can use this information when drafting the high-level solution design and description.

Thank you for your time today. These results will help the task force develop a high-level solution design for the purposes of developing and costing a five-year strategy and one-year road map. Once the draft is developed, members from senior management will be called to a steering committee or technical working group to discuss and validate the design. [Note: The facilitator should give a time frame, if available, for next steps.]

ANNEX 4B. TELEMEDICINE OR HEALTH HOTLINE SERVICES UPTAKE ASSESSMENT TOOL

Purpose: The Telemedicine or Health Hotline Services Uptake Assessment Tool helps governments understand the individual and structural factors, as well as characteristics of the intervention, that may affect uptake of telemedicine or health hotline services. This assessment prepares the government to select a solution that leverages opportunities and mitigates any anticipated challenges. The tool consists of three parts:

1. Interviews with community members tool
2. Interviews with health workers tool
3. Government reflection guide

Timing: This assessment should be completed after the government has conducted brief prescoping to confirm and describe the need for telemedicine or health hotline services.

Instructions: The focal point leading the drive—or another a person or organization identified by the focal point—should (1) conduct interviews with community members targeted to use the service and with health care workers and (2) facilitate a reflection session with the government task force.

The interview sampling design should consider the following:

Community interviews	Health worker interviews
• Urban, periurban, and rural areas • Demographics (age and gender) • Geographic distribution within the country • Socioeconomic background • Culture, religion, and language	• Health system level (community, health center, district hospital, and so on) • Demographics (age and gender) • Geographic distribution within the country

Monitoring and evaluation specialists within the ministry of health should advise on sampling size depending on the funding available and the extent of variability within the target population. For example, if the target population is relatively homogeneous in terms of religion, language, and culture, a smaller sample size may be acceptable. Interviews can be conducted with individuals or in focus groups of approximately eight respondents per group. If some or all of the interviews will be conducted in focus groups, the evaluation design should consider the willingness of participants to speak openly in a mixed group versus in a group of their peers. For example, it is typically best to hold separate focus groups for men and women. In addition, focus groups with community leaders or health workers should not include community members and vice versa.

When deciding whether to conduct interviews or focus groups, keep in mind that facilitating focus groups requires special skills to encourage participation and capture differing viewpoints. Collecting high-quality data should be valued above collecting a high number of interviews; 25 individual interviews with rich data and honest discussion are better than focus group discussions with 100 respondents who did not feel comfortable participating.

Governments should adapt these tools to the context, including translation as needed.

1. Interviews with community members

Introduction: The interviewer should start with a personal introduction and an explanation of the assessment, such as the following:

Hello, my name is [__]. I represent [name of organization and one sentence explaining what this organization does]. I am talking to community members on behalf of the government to learn about how people in this community access health information and medical treatment to inform potential new services such as telemedicine or health hotlines. Our conversation should last less than 30 minutes. We are talking to many people, and we will summarize the conversations for the government; however, your name will remain anonymous. We will audio record the conversation to make sure we capture everything. Are you willing to participate in the interview?

Is now a convenient time to talk?

If the person is not willing to participate or it is not a convenient time, thank the person for his or her time. If the person is willing, continue.

Date of interview: _____

Number of respondents: _____

Gender of respondents: _____

Location: _____

Question	Answer
1. What do you do if you have questions about your health or your family's health? Whom do you ask or where do you go?	
a. Can you give me an example of when you have done this?	
b. How confident are you in the health information you receive?	
c. Do you have any challenges finding the information you need about your health or your family's health? If so, what are those challenges?	
2. What do you currently do when you or a family member shows symptoms of illness?	
a. Can you give me an example of when you did that?	
b. How confident are you in the treatment you receive in this way?	
c. Do you have any challenges finding the information you need about your health or your family's health? If so, what are those challenges?	

continued

Question	Answer
3. Do you personally own a mobile phone? Is it a basic feature phone or a smartphone?	
a. If not, do you have access to a mobile phone in another way? If yes, what way? What kind of phone is it—a basic feature phone or a smartphone?	
b. Do you currently use your mobile phone or the mobile phone you can access to [insert activities relevant to the technology under consideration, such as make voice calls, send Short Message Service messages, send messages through WhatsApp, or others]?	
4. [Health hotline] Would you be comfortable using a mobile phone to get reliable answers to questions about your health or your family's health? Why or why not?	
a. Do you think there are any benefits to doing this?	
b. Do you have any concerns about doing this?	
Allow the respondent to answer. Then ask:	
i. Would you have any concerns about confidentiality? Why or why not?	
ii. Would you have any concerns if this service worked just like any voice call and cost airtime? Why or why not?	
iii. Would you have any concerns if the service required sending messages through WhatsApp and used data airtime? Why or why not?	
c. How confident would you be in the health information you received in this way?	
d. Do you think that using a mobile phone to call a hotline would be a better, similar, or worse way to access information about your health? Why?	
e. Do you recommend that the government offer a hotline like this? Why or why not?	
5. [Telemedicine] Would you be comfortable using a mobile phone to consult a health care worker for treatment for a medical condition or problem? Why or why not?	
a. Do you think there are any benefits to doing this?	

continued

Question	Answer
b. Do you have any concerns about doing this?	
c. How confident would you be in the treatment you received in this way?	
d. Do you think that using a mobile phone to consult a health care worker for treatment would be a better, similar, or worse way to access treatment? Why?	
e. Do you recommend that the government offer a service to access treatment like this? Why or why not?	
6. Where do you hear about new programs or services in your community?	
a. What other ways do people in your community hear about new programs or services?	
b. Do you have suggestions for how to share information about new programs and services with the community?	
7. Do you have anything else to share about accessing health information or treatment?	

Thank you for your valuable time and input. The information you have given the government will help it make strategic decisions about new health care services.

2. Interviews with health workers

Introduction: The interviewer should start with a personal introduction and an explanation of the assessment, such as the following:

Hello, my name is [__]. I represent [name of organization and one sentence explaining what this organization does]. I am talking to community members on behalf of the government to learn about how people in this community access health information and medical treatment to inform potential new services such as telemedicine or health hotlines. Our conversation should last less than 30 minutes. We are talking to many people, and we will summarize the conversations for the government; however, your name will remain anonymous. We will audio record the conversation to make sure we capture everything. Are you willing to participate in the interview?

Is now a convenient time to talk?

If the person is not willing to participate or it is not a convenient time, thank the person for his or her time. If the person is willing, continue.

Date of interview: _____

Gender of respondents: _____

Health system level: _____

Location: _____

Question	Answer
1. What do people in this community do when they have a question about their health? Whom do they ask or where do they go?	
a. Do you think this is sufficient for them to get the information they are looking for? Why or why not?	
b. Do you think that people in this community have any challenges finding the information they need? If so, what are those challenges?	
2. What do people in this community do when they show symptoms of illness?	
a. Do you think this is sufficient for them to receive the treatment they need? Why or why not?	
b. Do you think people in this community have any challenges getting the treatment they need? If so, what are those challenges?	
3. What do you do if you have a medical question about how to help the people you are serving and your supervisor is not present? Whom do you ask or what do you do? How do you access this resource?	
a. Can you give me an example of when you have done this?	
b. How satisfied are you with the information you receive in this way? Why?	
c. Do you have any challenges finding information in this way so that you can provide medical care? What are those challenges?	
4. What do you do if a patient needs to access specialist care that is not available at your health facility?	
a. Can you give me an example of when this occurred?	
b. How satisfied are you with this method? Why?	
c. Are there any challenges accessing specialist care in this way? If so, what are those challenges?	
5. Do you personally own a mobile phone? Is this a basic feature phone or a smartphone?	
a. If not, do you have access to a mobile phone in another way? If yes, what way? What kind of phone is it—a basic feature phone or a smartphone?	

continued

Question	Answer
b. Do you currently use your mobile phone or the mobile phone you can access to [insert activities relevant to the technology under consideration, such as make voice calls, send Short Message Service messages, send messages through WhatsApp, or others]?	
6. Have you heard of health hotlines, in which people call a number to ask trained operators their health questions? If yes, what have you heard about health hotlines?	
a. Do you think that this would be an effective way for people in your community to get information about their health? Why or why not?	
b. Would you feel comfortable providing advice to people in your community by mobile phone? Why or why not?	
c. Do you think health hotlines would be an effective way for you to get answers to your medical questions? Why or why not?	
d. Do you have any concerns about getting answers to your medical questions this way? What are they?	
e. Do you think that using a mobile phone to call a hotline would be a better, similar, or worse way to access the information you need? Why?	
f. Do you recommend that the government introduce a health hotline, either for the community or to support health workers? Why or why not?	
7. Have you heard of telemedicine, in which people use their mobile phones to consult a health care worker for treatment for a medical condition or problem? If yes, what have you heard about telemedicine?	
a. Do you think that this would be an effective way for people in your community to access treatment? Why or why not?	
b. Would you feel comfortable offering medical treatment by mobile phone? Why or why not?	
c. Do you think telemedicine would be an effective way for you to access specialist services for your patients? Why or why not?	

continued

Question	Answer
d. Do you have any concerns about accessing a specialist in this way? What are they?	
e. Do you think telemedicine would be a better, similar, or worse way to access specialist services for your patients? Why?	
f. Do you recommend that the government introduce a mobile phone service to consult either a health care worker or specialist for treatment? Why or why not?	
8. Do you have anything else to share about accessing health information or treatment?	

Thank you for your valuable time and input. The information you have given the government will help it make strategic decisions about new health care services.

3. Government reflection guide

Instructions: Data from the two tools drafted before should be transcribed, analyzed, and summarized for presentation, potentially via PowerPoint, to the relevant government task force. When analyzing the data, the analysis team should consider the following:

- Where is there consensus among respondents?
- Where do differences exist between groups (community members versus health workers, male community members versus female community members, community health workers versus health workers at district hospitals, and so on)?
- Even if they are not a majority view, are there critical questions or issues that exist among a minority of respondents?

List the following data:

Number of respondents: _____

Gender of respondents: _____

Location: _____

Individual and behavioral characteristics

1. [Patient needs and resources] Thinking about data on **community members' current resources for health information and treatment**, did anything surprise you?
    a. Which groups seem to have the greatest need for access to health information? For access to health treatment? What evidence do you have?
    b. Do health workers seem to understand the behavior and needs of their patients? What evidence do you have?

2. [Tension for change] Thinking about the **challenges that community members experience**, did anything surprise you?
    a. Does the need for health hotlines and telemedicine seem urgent and critical overall? What evidence do you have?
    b. Were there any groups for whom the need is particularly urgent? What evidence do you have?

3. [Knowledge and beliefs about intervention] Thinking about data on **perceptions of health hotlines and telemedicine**, did anything surprise you?

   a. What were the most common benefits that respondents expressed? Are these benefits likely to be achieved by the intervention?

   b. Did any groups express concern about using health hotlines? What were their concerns? Did any groups express concern about using telemedicine? What were their concerns? How did these concerns differ?

   c. Did any groups mention language barriers, low literacy rates, or socioeconomic factors as concerns in accessing health hotlines or telemedicine? What were these concerns?

Structural or practical characteristics

4. [Networks and communications] Thinking about data on **mobile phone access**, did anything surprise you?

   a. Is mobile phone coverage sufficient for the introduction of a health hotline? What evidence do you have?

   b. Is smartphone coverage sufficient for the introduction of telemedicine? What evidence do you have?

5. [External policies and incentives] Thinking about data on **sources of information about new programs**, did anything surprise you?

   a. What are the most common resources? Do these resources differ between community members and health workers? What evidence do you have?

Intervention characteristics

6. [Relative advantage] Thinking about data on **recommendations and comparisons to other options**, did anything surprise you?

   a. Did respondents express any alternative interventions to address the needs? What were they? Which groups identified them?

   b. Did any groups not recommend that the government offer health hotlines? Why not? Did any group think the government should not offer telemedicine? Why not? How did these recommendations differ?

ANNEX 4C. LANDSCAPE ANALYSIS TOOL: QUESTIONNAIRE AND ANALYSIS REFLECTION GUIDE FOR GOVERNMENT AND STAKEHOLDERS

Purpose: This landscape analysis helps governments understand what existing telemedicine, hotline, and related services exist in the country. The government may choose someone from inside the government or an external consultant to conduct the landscape analysis and questionnaire. This landscape analysis helps governments build on what already exists and develop a plan for coordination and interoperability between the various services and partners. This tool consists of three parts:

1. Interview questionnaire for government officials
2. Interview questionnaire for other stakeholders
3. Government analysis reflection guide

Note: A government may choose to use the same questions for both government and other stakeholders and can choose to use the interview questions listed or adapt the questions for its purposes.

Timing: This assessment should be completed after the government has conducted prescoping of the solution and has assessed potential uptake of the services.

Instructions: The focal point leading the planning for telemedicine or health hotline services should identify (if not doing it personally) a person or organization to (1) conduct interviews with critical stakeholders and (2) facilitate a reflection session with the government small task force and steering committee or technical working group.

The interviews should start with a known list of interested government department focal points and service providers in the country. The interviewer would then expand the list using a chain-referral sampling methodology based on the recommendations from the interviewees. Note that stakeholders listed in this matrix are based on the official titles of the Malawi stakeholders involved in the Chipatala Cha Pa Foni, or Health Center by Phone, solution. Each government has different titles and structures and will need to adapt the titles as relevant.

Government interviews	Other stakeholders

Ministry of Health:
 	
• Directorate of Clinical Services
• Directorate of Preventive Health Services
  – Health Education Services
  – Community Health
• Department of Planning and Policy Development—Digital Health Division
• Department of Information and Communication Technology
• External Partnerships Division (if it exists)
• Departments related to specific health topics (as relevant): maternal, newborn, and child health; sexual and reproductive services; Expanded Programme on Immunization; nutrition; noncommunicable diseases; tuberculosis; malaria; and so on
• Medical specialty departments: dermatology, mental health, and so on
	• Mobile network operators
	• Donors that may be funding current services
	
	Service providers of:
	• Telemedicine
	• Hotlines
	• Interactive voice response, Unstructured Supplementary Service Data, or WhatsApp services that might be integrated

The following tools should be adapted to the country context, including translation as needed.

1. Interview questionnaire for government officials

Introduction (5 minutes): The interviewer should start with a personal introduction and an explanation of the assessment, such as the following:

Hello, my name is [__]. I represent [name of organization and one sentence explaining what this organization does] to better understand the current telemedicine or health hotline landscape in [insert country name]. The government will use this information to build on what already exists and develop a plan for coordination and interoperability between the various services and partners. [If applicable: Thank you for the materials that you provided in advance of this conversation. They were helpful to us and have allowed us to streamline our questions today.] Do you have any questions before we get started? [Answer any questions.] We are talking to many people, and we will summarize the conversations for the government; however, your name will remain anonymous. We will audio record the conversation to make sure we capture everything. Are you willing to participate in the interview?

[If the interviewee is willing, press record.]

Questions the interviewee asks the interviewer: _____

Name of interviewer: _____

Name of interviewee: _____

Organization and title of interviewee: _____

Date of interview: _____

Q #	Question	Response
Existing hotlines and messaging services and mobile network provider information in _____ [name of country] Greens are must haves. Blacks are nice to have.		
Background		
1.	What is your position in the government?	
2.	How are you involved in managing or creating policy for telemedicine or health hotlines or other health care services more broadly? • Are there other government agencies to manage telemedicine or health hotlines? • Are there other government agencies that should be involved? • Is there any coordination on telemedicine or health hotlines across the different governments within [name of country] currently?	

continued

Q #	Question	Response
Service delivery		
3.	Does the country have any existing public or free telemedicine or health hotline services?	
4.	Given what you know about the (public or private) telemedicine or health hotline services offered in [name of country] currently • How are your office or other government agencies working with these service providers? • What is your perception of the quality of these services? • In your opinion, how well does the current scope of the services (geographic reach and type of services) meet the need?	
5.	Are you working with these service providers to address gaps or incorporate any new services? • Are any of these planned services specialty care services (that is, nonprimary care)?	
6.	How are the telemedicine or health hotline services currently helping to address needs due to the COVID-19 pandemic?	
User needs		
7.	Have you or anyone you know of completed any evaluation or assessment of needs for telemedicine or health hotlines in [name of country]? • If yes, are you able to share the results?	
8.	Are there other common health issues not being addressed by telemedicine or health hotlines that you think should be addressed? Why? • What are the most appropriate topics and specialties for telemedicine in [name of country] in your opinion? Why?	
9.	What do you see as the main opportunities for telemedicine or health hotlines to address the health needs of the [name of country] people?	
10.	How do you see telemedicine or health hotlines helping in addressing any other needs of the [name of country] government?	

continued

Q #	Question	Response
Current usage		
11.	Do you monitor the use of telemedicine or health hotline services? How? • How many people use the telemedicine or health hotline service every month? • Do you know the demographics of the individuals who use the service? • Do you have a dashboard and way of monitoring the service volume, scope, breadth, and so on of health topics? If yes, what other information does it include? • Are there groups you feel are not being reached by the service?	
12.	Do you feel the existing health system (hospitals, clinics, and so on) can address the needs identified through the telemedicine or health hotline program? For example, can someone identified as having a mental health crisis receive the appropriate follow-up services?	
13.	Do you promote the use of telemedicine or health hotline services? If so, how?	
14.	[If applicable] How has the public reacted to the availability of telehealth or health hotline services for COVID-19 and primary health services?	
Organizational issues		
15.	What legal and reimbursement standards, if any, does the government provide to support the implementation of telemedicine or health hotline service?	
16.	How do you ensure that service providers adhere to the legal and regulatory policies of the country?	
17.	Are there legal or regulatory policies that you think should exist that do not?	
18.	How would you describe the government's ability to financially support expanding or strengthening telemedicine or health hotline services?	
19.	Has the government identified any official goals or targets for expanding or strengthening telemedicine or health hotline services?	
20.	Are telemedicine or health hotline services already built into the health sector strategic plans and budgets?	

continued

Q #	Question	Response
Technology		
21.	In your opinion, is the technology infrastructure in [name of country] sufficient to provide the level and type of telemedicine or health hotline services that you would like to see? • If not, what are the main barriers in your opinion? • Does [name of country] experience power supply issues? If so, how regularly?	
22.	What is the level of smartphone coverage in the country?	
23.	Do people without smartphones have other avenues for getting health information by phone?	
24.	[If applicable] If not, what do you see as the priorities for improving technology infrastructure?	
25.	Does the government have any official goals or targets for improving technology infrastructure?	
26.	Do you have any questions about the type of technologies and infrastructure required or that would benefit [name of country] to implement telemedicine or health hotline services?	
27.	Do you have any questions related to data security or housing servers? If so, what are those questions?	
28.	Do you have an agreement of any sort with mobile network operators? If so, with whom?	
Challenges and future plans		
29.	What are the biggest challenges that the government faces in managing and building up telemedicine or health hotline services to meet the country's health needs? • Does the biggest need relate to people, process, resources, or technology?	
30.	What type of information or support do you think would best help the government to strengthen or grow the telemedicine or health hotline services in [name of country]?	
31.	What additional needs or opportunities could the telemedicine service resolve (for example, training opportunities or network collaboration with specialized providers, such as communities of practice)?	
32.	Is there anything else you would like us to know about the current telemedicine or health hotline landscape or [name of country]'s needs around it?	

continued

Q #	Question	Response
33.	Do you know of any other people we should contact? If so, please provide the contact information.	
34.	Do you have any other questions for us?	

Thank you for your valuable time and input. The information you have given the government will help it build upon and coordinate what exists for an integrated health system.

2.   Interview questionnaire for other stakeholders

Primary objectives (for interviewer knowledge):

1. Determine what telemedicine, health hotlines, and messaging services exist within the country and what they provide.
2. Determine preliminary interest and additional need for telemedicine or health hotline services.
3. Determine next steps for coordination with the government.

Introduction (5 minutes): The interviewer should start with a personal introduction and an explanation of the assessment, such as the following:

Hello, my name is [__]. I represent [name of organization and one sentence explaining what this organization does] to better understand the current telemedicine or health hotline landscape in [insert country name]. The government will use this information to build on what already exists and develop a plan for coordination and interoperability between the systems and partners. [If applicable: Thank you for the materials that you provided in advance of this conversation. They were helpful to us and have allowed us to streamline our questions today.] Do you have any questions before we get started? [Answer any questions.] We are talking to many people, and we will summarize the conversations for the government; however, your name will remain anonymous. We will audio record the conversation to make sure we capture everything. Are you willing to participate in the interview?

[If the interviewee is willing, press record.]

Questions the interviewee asks the interviewer: _____

Name of interviewer: _____

Name of interviewee: _____

Organization and title of interviewee: _____

Type of interviewee [government, potential partner, donor, other stakeholder]: _____

Date of interview: _____

#	Question	Answer
	Existing hotlines and messaging services and mobile network provider information in _____ **[name of country]** Interviewer note: If you are interviewing implementers of a known hotline or messaging service, you can ask them question 2 first and then ask if they know about others and the details of those. **Greens** are must haves. **Blacks** are nice to have. (Time: 30 minutes)	
1.	While we have done some research on services in the country, to your knowledge, are there (other) telemedicine, health hotline, or messaging services in the country that are well used? [Ask if they know several so you can plan interview accordingly.] • If yes, ask for the name of the service. • No (unknown) • *Specify the criteria for which we are looking: Is the service health-focused, is it larger than simply a pilot program, is it government endorsed*	
2.	For any that exist please answer the following questions: [Interviewers use matrix to fill in information.] 1. Ownership/Stewardship: Can you please describe the following? a. Who operates the service? b. Who are the key decision-makers for the service? i. Government ii. Partner: _____ iii. Other: _____ c. How is the government involved (if at all)? Does the government support (not necessarily financially) or back the services (is it in line with the government strategic objectives)? i. Yes. [Follow up by asking, In what way does the government support the service?] ii. No iii. Unknown 2. Scope: Please describe the topics it covers (open-ended). a. All health b. Maternal, newborn, and child health c. Family planning d. Adolescent e. HIV/AIDS f. Other: _____ 3. Does the service only provide health information, or is it also diagnostic? Does it provide referrals to secondary or tertiary centers? 4. Does the service follow up with the caller (in person or through callbacks) after a specified period? If yes, please explain further. a. Yes b. No c. Unknown	

continued

#	Question	Answer
5.	If it is a messaging service, does it send out public service announcements to all users or targeted users, such as through notification of immunization campaigns on specific dates and in specific areas? If yes, please explain further. a. Yes b. No c. Unknown d. Not applicable	
6.	Technology: a. Please describe how that service is administered and what technology is used. [Probe on Short Message Service, WhatsApp, hotline, Unstructured Supplementary Service Data, and so on.] b. Data storage: What is the government's policy on health data storage? (For example, other governments do not allow offshore data storage.) How do other health hotlines store data? c. Systems integration: What is the government's policy or strategy around e-health systems integration?	
7.	Mobile network operators: a. Which mobile operators does the service use, if any? What is the government's relationship with that provider? Do you know if there is an agreement with the operator for reduced or zero-rated costs? b. Do you know if the mobile network operators allow unregistered Short Message Service or blast campaigns? If yes, please explain. i. Yes ii. No iii. Unknown	
8.	Coverage: a. What geographic range does the service cover (district names, nationwide, etc.)? For how long has it operated at that scale? b. Do certain populations (such as urban, rural, migrants, refugees, etc.) mostly use it? If yes, please explain. i. Yes ii. No iii. Unknown	
9.	Monitoring/Quality Assurance: Do you know what monitoring and evaluation indicators the service tracks, or what quality assurance measures are put in place and how that information is shared and used? If yes, please explain. a. Yes b. No c. Unknown	
10.	Financing: a. Are any costs incurred by the end user for using the service? b. Who pays for the service currently? c. If different, who will pay for the service in the long run (government, donor, private, or a combination)? d. Is this service covered under the national health insurance scheme (if one exists)? If yes, please explain. i. Yes ii. No iii. Unknown iv. Does not exist	

continued

#	Question	Answer
	11. Is the service subscription-only and only available to specific communities? Please specify. a. Yes b. No c. Unknown 12. Scale and Sustainability: What are the plans for the hotline in the next 5–10 years? a. Are there plans for scaling it up programmatically or geographically, if it is not already nationwide? If yes, please explain. i. Yes ii. No iii. Unknown b. In your view, how will the service be financially sustainable long term? 13. Contact: Do you know a contact for the service, and if so, can we please have a contact name and email? a. Yes b. No	
	**Need and interest to upgrade existing systems and desired capabilities (if applicable)** (Time: 10 minutes)	
3.	If applicable, what gaps exist in the current services? Please give examples, such as the ability to serve the population, sustainability plans, and so on.	
	**Need and interest for a service similar to telemedicine or a health hotline (if applicable)** (Time: 10 minutes)	
4.	[If a telemedicine or combination hotline/messaging service does not exist] Do you feel there is a need and interest in the country? Why or why not? Please provide an example.	
5.	If yes, would this solution be in line with the current ministry of health strategic plans and priorities? 1. What topics should it cover? 2. Who would be the primary audience? [Open-ended, but interviewer should check as applicable.] a. Community b. Adolescents c. Health care workers d. Community health care workers e. Migrants f. Refugees g. Urban poor h. Other: _____ 3. What types of services should be offered? [Open-ended, but interviewer should check as applicable.] a. Hotline b. WhatsApp c. Tailored voice or Short Message Service messages	

continued

#	Question	Answer
	d. Outbreak surveillance e. Feedback loops on quality of service f. Links to emergency transport g. Diagnostic capabilities on specialized health topics h. Other: _____	
Avenues for moving a telemedicine or health hotline (Time: 5 minutes)		
6.	If we find there is interest in this type of service, we will plan in-person visits and work with the government to call together key stakeholders to discuss it. Whom do you recommend we interview? Do technical working groups or other consortiums exist that might be worth incorporating when planning a stakeholder session (whether presenting and discussing at existing meetings or asking those groups to help coordinate with their members)? If so, please name them.	
7.	What other advice do you have for moving forward on this type of service (if that is what you recommend)?	
Other questions or other contacts (Time: 5 minutes)		
8.	Do you know of any other people we should contact? If so, please provide the contact information.	
9.	Do you have any other questions for us?	

Thank you so much for taking the time to talk to us today. We really appreciate it. Can we reach out with any follow-up questions? We will keep you posted on next steps and hope to talk to you again in the future.

3. Government analysis reflection guide

Instructions: Data from the two tools drafted before should be transcribed, analyzed, and summarized for presentation to the relevant government task force. See the Terms of Reference for the Telemedicine or Health Hotline Planning Task Force (annex 3A) and the Terms of Reference for Telemedicine or Health Hotline Multisector Steering Committee (annex 5A). When analyzing the data, the analysis team should consider the following:

- Where is there consensus among respondents?
- Are there services that multiple people are aware of, and how do the operations and advertising of those services differ?
- Could the government partner with some of the existing service providers or help scale those services by embedding them into the public sector?
- What recommendations could the government use in its solution design for telemedicine or health hotline services?

The data collection team lead could present the data using PowerPoint to facilitate discussion.

Number of respondents: _____

Number of government respondents: _____

Number of potential nongovernmental organization partner respondents: _____

Number of potential private sector respondents: _____

Number of donors: _____

Landscape Analysis Results Matrix

The interviewer or analyst can populate the following table according to the results of the interviews. This matrix can help the government quickly interpret what opportunities for partnership and growth related to telemedicine or health hotline services exist in the country.

#	Name of existing service	Service operator or owner	Type of service (telemedicine, hotline, Short Message Service, Unstructured Supplementary Service Data, WhatsApp)	Health scope	Target population	Current network operators the service uses	Current scale	Perceived or documented current quality or impact of service	Plans for expansion or integration into the public sector	Recommendations for improving or expanding services

ANNEX 4D. TELEMEDICINE OR HEALTH HOTLINE SOLUTION DESIGN DECISION-MAKING TOOL

Purpose: The Telemedicine or Health Hotline Solution Design Decision-Making Tool helps governments answer the critical questions needed for solution design to then move forward on costing and planning.

Timing: The planning task force should complete this table after the government has determined the following:

- Political stability
- Technical requirements
- Health areas of greatest need
- Target audience of the solution
- Potential uptake of the services
- Landscape of existing services

Instructions: The planning task force should convene and come to a consensus on the answers in this tool based on the previous discussions with government officials and results from the scoping, targeting, and landscape analyses.

#	Decision-making question	Possible answers	Considerations
1.	Given smartphone coverage and the ability of the population to use audio or video, which type of service does the government want to move forward with at this time?	• Telemedicine • Health hotline	
2a.	Given information from the prescoping exercise, which health areas does the government want the service to cover immediately (in the next 3–12 months)?	Assign a number based on priority to the following, and leave blank if the government will not cover the topic in the next 3–6 months. • COVID-19 • Maternal, newborn, and child health (includes vaccination) • Sexual and reproductive health • HIV • Infectious diseases • Noncommunicable diseases • Mental health • Other: _____ • Specialty services (applicable only to telemedicine). List specific services: _____	The government may not be able to cover all health topics in 12 months if building it out, but it may if using existing services. It is important to prioritize.

continued

#	Decision-making question	Possible answers	Considerations
2b.	Which health areas does the government want the service to cover within the next five years?	• All primary health topics (if chosen, prioritize with numbers) • COVID-19 (including vaccine information) • Maternal, newborn, and child health (includes vaccination) • Sexual and reproductive health • HIV • Infectious diseases • Noncommunicable diseases • Mental health • Other: _____ • Specialty services (applicable only to telemedicine). List specific services: _____	This answer is critical because the solution should be designed for the desired scale to optimize investment.

3a.	Who is the target audience in the next 3–12 months?	• Health care workers
		  – List cadres below:
		  _____
		• Direct to consumer (community)
			The target audience for direct to consumer may be further defined by the health coverage area. For example, maternal, newborn, and child health might target expecting mothers and parents (including fathers) of children.

3b.	Who is the target audience in the next five years?	• Health care workers
		  – List cadres below:
		  _____
		• Direct to consumer (community)	

4.	Does the government plan to use an existing service for immediate setup?	• Yes
		  – List service (partner) below:
		  _____
		• No
		• Unknown
			If this is unknown or dependent on costing, the task force may have to provide both options to the steering committee. Whether the answer is yes or no, further information will be required for the cost modeling. See Telemedicine or Health Hotline Cost Model Tool (annex 9A).

continued

#	Decision-making question	Possible answers	Considerations
4a.	If yes, is the plan to outsource now and embed in the future, or will the service be outsourced for the foreseeable future but eventually embedded in the government plans and budgets?	• Outsource now only and embed in the future • Outsource for the foreseeable future, but the government would pay these outsourcing costs • Unknown	May require further discussion in the five-year strategy session.
5.	Whether the service is outsourced or not, what is the minimum cadre that is acceptable for the services according to existing regulations?	• Non-health worker trained on frequently asked questions only • Community health worker • Nurses • Clinical officers • Physicians • Physicians with specialties (telemedicine only) • Unknown; needs further discussion	The task force may propose this critical decision, but ultimately the steering committee or technical working group would decide.
6.	Will the service be free to users?	• Yes • No	
6a.	If yes, how will the government pay for the cost of the incoming calls?	• Direct payment by government or through donor or partner • Already established agreement with mobile network operator • Planned agreement with mobile network operator	Sustainable solutions that governments can afford will require reduced or zero-rated costs from mobile network operators in the country.

7.	Does the government plan to use other technologies integrated into the telemedicine or health hotline services in the next five years?	• Yes
		  – Interactive voice response
		  – WhatsApp
		  – Short Message Service
		  – Unstructured Supplementary Service Data
		  – Other: _____
		• No
		• Unknown
			Using additional technologies can help meet demand.

The five-year strategy session is where the high-level steering committee will make the critical decisions, but this tool helps establish initial design.

NOTES

1. The Uptake Assessment Tool uses key aspects of the Consolidated Framework for Implementation Research, a well-established source for implementation of science research—see the "Updated CFIR Constructs" web page (https://cfirguide.org /constructs/).
2. See the World Health Organization's Digital Health Atlas (https://digitalhealthatlas.org /en/-/) or Digital Impact Alliance's Catalog of Digital Solutions (https://solutions.dial .community/products) for a range of digital technologies and partners that may help with telemedicine, health hotline, or related technologies in the country.

REFERENCE

PAHO (Pan American Health Organization) and IDB (Inter-American Development Bank). 2020. "COVID-19 and Telemedicine: Tool for Assessing the Maturity Level of Health Institutions to Implement Telemedicine Services." Version 3.0, PAHO, Washington, DC. https://www3.paho.org/ish/images/toolkit/COVID-19-Telemedicine_RATool-en.pdf?ua=1.

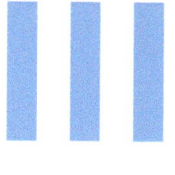

Develop Strategy, Implementation Road Map, and Budget

During Phase 2, the government will align on the vision it wants to achieve, preliminarily plan for implementation, and determine the cost of the proposed solution strategy and road map. Each of these actions is needed to plan for sustainability from the outset.

- Chapter 5 helps governments understand how to align on the vision they hope to achieve through a five-year strategy.
- Chapter 6 helps governments develop a private sector strategy.
- Chapter 7 details development of the one-year road map that the government will use for implementation planning.
- Chapter 8 helps the government better understand the many technical and service provider aspects of planning for and ultimately implementing telemedicine or health hotline services.
- Chapter 9 helps governments cost the solution, strategy, and road map. After validating these elements, the government can then begin Phases 3 and 4: securing funding for start-up and for establishing, implementing, scaling, and sustaining telemedicine or health hotline services in the country.

Establish a Steering Committee and Develop a Five-Year Strategy for Setting Up, Implementing, and Operating and Managing Telemedicine or Health Hotline Services

Chapter 5 helps the government align on the vision it hopes to achieve. The government does so by first establishing a decision-making steering committee to validate the initial solution design, by ensuring regulatory compliance from the outset, and by developing a five-year strategy. This chapter presents the following tools:

- *Terms of Reference for Telemedicine or Health Hotline Multisector Steering Committee (annex 5A)*
- *Telemedicine or Health Hotline Five-Year Strategy Decision-Making Tool (annex 5B)*
- *Sample Telemedicine or Health Hotline Five-Year Strategy (annex 5C)*

ESTABLISH A MULTISECTOR STEERING COMMITTEE AND VALIDATE THE BASIC SOLUTION DESIGN

The multisector steering committee[1] provides ultimate decision-making authority and oversight for planning and establishing the services, as well as for ongoing monitoring, coordinating stakeholders, and embedding the solution into the public sector. Whereas the planning task force produces materials for review, a steering committee ultimately discusses and signs off on solution design. The lead department at the ministry of health that will be operating the service should chair the steering committee, which should have members from multiple ministry of health departments and representatives from health regulatory bodies, the ministry of finance, the ministry of justice, and the ministry of communication; relevant mobile network operators (MNOs); a range of service providers; national health sciences research committees; and other relevant partners as needed. See the detailed Terms of Reference for Telemedicine or Health Hotline Multisector Steering Committee in annex 5A.

The planning task force should present all the initial findings from tools in Phases 0 and 1 and then offer an initial solution design for discussion and validation. Because many steering committee members will have provided input into the initial Telemedicine or Health Hotline Predesign Scoping (annex 4A), Uptake Assessment (annex 4B), Landscape Analysis (annex 4C), and Solution Design (annex 4D), achieving alignment should not be difficult; however, it is necessary to document the validation and ultimately receive sign-off from the highest decision-making authority, likely the minister of health or secretary for health, before moving forward with further planning. This validation meeting may take two to three hours depending on the decision-makers' level of alignment going into the meeting.

ENSURE COMPLIANCE WITH REGULATORY BODIES FROM THE OUTSET

As noted in the Stakeholder Matrix (annex 3B) and the Steering Committee Terms of Reference (annex 5A), the government should include regulatory bodies from both health and communications in critical discussions and decision-making from the outset. To ensure compliance, these regulatory bodies should have an appointed focal point for the steering committee throughout the process. For already established hotline services, the government will need to assess that the service provider is registered (if applicable) and adheres to the current in-country regulations. If the government does not have scope of practice or health data governance regulations related to telemedicine or health hotline services, the steering committee should include the health and communications regulatory bodies to guide drafting those regulations. The drafting of regulations is out of scope for this toolkit.

DEVELOP A TELEMEDICINE OR HEALTH HOTLINE FIVE-YEAR STRATEGY

Both telemedicine and hotline services can be set up quickly, but for sustainability the government should develop, at the start, a five-year strategy that outlines goals and objectives for each year. Based on the solution validation, the steering committee should define the vision for what the solution will achieve over five years. In the predesign scoping, the ministry of health will have already determined what health areas and services it ultimately wants, but it may choose a phased approach for service delivery. The strategy consists of five main aspects:

1. *Solution management:* who will manage the solution each year, including technology upgrades (management may change from a service provider to coleading to government)
2. *Solution impact or outcome:* what outcomes the government hopes to see (they may change from basic service outcomes preliminarily to impact indicators once the service has operated for a couple of years)
3. *Health areas:* which health areas the service will serve

4. *Services:* what services will be offered (telemedicine, hotline, voices messages, Short Message Service, WhatsApp, and the like)
5. *Geographic coverage:* what areas of the country the service will reach

The Telemedicine or Health Hotline Five-Year Strategy Decision-Making Tool (annex 5B) provides the questions that must be answered to align on the government's vision. Answers to each question should be provided for each year. The focal point with the planning task force can help facilitate development of this five-year strategy, but the steering committee with high-level decision-makers must provide input and ultimately approve the strategy in writing. The tool itself should take the focal point and planning task force only an hour to fill out but requires discussions with government officials over a period of one to two weeks, depending on availability. As previously noted, the actual validation should happen at a steering committee meeting that would take two to three hours because it would include presentation of all information that fed into the solution design. See also the Sample Telemedicine or Health Hotline Five-Year Strategy in annex 5C.

The five-year strategy provides the foundation for all other planning. Without a solid five-year strategy, the government will find it difficult to build requests for proposals from service providers, create a one-year road map, or budget for the first five years.

Ensure integration of this system into the service delivery structure so that it doesn't become a silo of care. This telemedicine or health hotline should be integrated into the current health care system, for example by referring patients to health centers; receiving and sending data to the patients' health centers; and communicating with other systems, such as laboratories, pharmacies, or community services.

ANNEX 5A. TERMS OF REFERENCE FOR TELEMEDICINE OR HEALTH HOTLINE MULTISECTOR STEERING COMMITTEE

Purpose: The purpose of the Terms of Reference for Telemedicine or Health Hotline Multisector Steering Committee is to help governments understand the goals, responsibilities, timing, and membership of the steering committee, which has the decision-making authority and oversight for the planning, establishment, ongoing monitoring, coordinating of stakeholders, and ultimate embedding of the nationwide, government-stewarded services in the country into the health system.

Timing: The government should form a steering committee after it has conducted all activities in Phases 0 and 1, including the initial solution design.

Instructions: The lead department at the ministry of health, which will operate the service, would chair this multisector steering committee and, at the first meeting, present the terms of reference so everyone can understand and agree on their roles. They will then continue with the responsibilities as laid out in the terms of reference.

INSERT COUNTRY X GOVERNMENT LOGO

TERMS OF REFERENCE FOR TELEMEDICINE OR HEALTH HOTLINE MULTISECTOR STEERING COMMITTEE

Purpose

The purpose of the [insert official title] is to provide ultimate decision-making authority and oversight for the planning, establishment, ongoing monitoring, coordinating of stakeholders, and ultimate embedding of the nationwide, government-stewarded [select: telemedicine, health hotline, or both telemedicine and health hotline] services in the country into the health system. The planning task force would produce materials for review, but this committee would ultimately discuss and sign off as a group.

The [insert the lead department at the ministry of health for the services] leads this multisector steering committee.

Specific responsibilities by phase

Phase 0: Assess basic requirements and express interest
Phase 1: Scope and design solution
Phase 2: Develop road map, implementation plan, and budget
Phase 3: Advocate for funding
Phase 4: Establish, implement, and scale

Phases 0–2

- Attend all called meetings. (Note: The meetings may not be at specific intervals in Phases 0–2 but will be individually called. Switching out members at regular meetings leads to delays and confusion.)
- Validate gap and landscape analysis presented by task force.
- Oversee the small task force to ensure progress on planning milestones.
- Provide individual and group input, and validate high-level scope and solution design and solution description for [select: national telemedicine or hotline] services, including guiding the decision-making process on staffing, location, supervision, training, and incorporation into strategic plans.
- Validate five-year strategy, including vision for implementation and ongoing sustainability and establishing key performance indicators, and validate one-year road map.
- Establish a subcommittee for partner selection to develop specific requests for proposals, review proposals, and select service providers (if applicable).
- Validate five-year strategy and one-year road map costs.
- Discuss options for, advocate for, and develop a plan for funding for [select: national telemedicine or hotline] services from respective government entities, donors, and partners.
- Develop a plan for any needed policy changes.
- Develop and validate an advertising and demand-generation plan for the services.

Phase 3

- Discuss options, advocate for, develop a plan, and assign roles for securing funding for [select: national telemedicine or hotline] services from respective government entities, donors, and partners.
- Discuss options, advocate, develop a plan, and assign roles for securing an agreement with the MNOs to provide short codes and zero-rate incoming calls (at minimum) and to advertise the service via free blasts (when allowable by the communications regulators in the specified country).

Phase 4

Governance and approval responsibilities

- Attend quarterly and relevant ad hoc meetings.
- Represent, advocate for, and support the development of [select: national telemedicine or hotline] services and support stakeholders' interests in the country.
- Coordinate other telemedicine or health hotline services in the country to ensure continuity of services if more than one exists in the country, and develop a road map for integration.
- Develop and enforce standardized guidelines and toolkits and policies for [select: national telemedicine or hotline] services.
- Advocate for and advise on [select: national telemedicine or hotline] technology development and applications, safety, and best practices.
- Validate or approve any critical plans or documents in accordance with the five-year strategy and one-year road map.

Establishment, implementation, and sustainability oversight responsibilities

- Validate an ongoing implementation and monitoring plan.
  - Review the data and key performance indicators at quarterly meetings, and provide feedback for how to improve services to meet needs and sustain impact.
- Oversee the establishment, implementation, scaling, and sustaining of the [select: national telemedicine or hotline] services.
  - Oversee the implementation of the sustainability plans (transition strategies, plans, readiness assessment), including ensuring that services get added to the ministry of health strategic plans and budgets.
  - Provide guidance and feedback on how to adjust plans if milestones and deliverables are not being met.
- Review any new [select: national telemedicine or hotline] implementer activity plans and activity reports for compliance to regulatory requirements; lessons sharing; and standardization of [select: national telemedicine or hotline] practices, research, and development.
- Provide risk management strategies, ensuring that strategies to address potential threats to the transition's success have been identified, estimated, and approved, and that the threats are regularly reassessed.

Regulatory responsibilities

- Review and provide advice on regulations to determine gaps and need for revision or updating.
- Coordinate with relevant sectors and ministries on the services' technology and safety.

Other responsibilities

- Promote and share technological development applications updates through invitation of various experts and organizations to present experiences to the steering committee or technical working group.
- Create a forum and information hub for sharing [select: national telemedicine or hotline] developments to general population.
- Set up subcommittees to pursue specific work streams as needed.
  - For example, regulatory subcommittee (sample terms of reference provided)
- Provide an annual review of the function of multisector [select: national telemedicine or hotline] [select: steering committee or technical working group] and adjust terms of reference accordingly.

Timing

The multisector [select: national telemedicine or hotline] steering committee will meet as needed (at least once per month) in Phases 0–2.

The multisector [select: national telemedicine or hotline] steering committee will meet quarterly in Phases 3–4 and will rotate support among its members.

Membership

The steering committee membership shall include the following. Department membership depends on the scope of the [select: national telemedicine or hotline] services provided. See the stakeholder matrix. Note that stakeholders listed in this matrix are based on the official titles of the Malawi stakeholders involved in the Chipatala Cha Pa Foni, or Health Center by Phone, solution. Because each government has different titles and structures, titles will need to be adapted as relevant.

- Ministry of Health
  - Directorate of Clinical Services (required)
  - Directorate of Preventive Health Services – Health Education Services (required)
  - Directorate of Preventive Health Services – Community Health Department (required)
  - Department of Planning and Policy Development (required)
  - Department of Planning and Policy Development – Central Monitoring and Evaluation Division (required)
  - Department of Planning and Policy Development – Quality Management Division (required)

- Department of Planning and Policy Development – Digital Health Division (required)
- Department of Information and Communication Technology (if country has one within the ministry of health and one for the government as a whole, the one in the ministry of health would be more relevant) (required)
- Department of Administration and Finance (in the Ministry of Health) (required)
- Department of Human Resources (required for in-house; may not be required out-of-house)
- Departments for specific health topics: maternal, newborn, and child health; sexual health and reproductive services; Expanded Programme on Immunization; nutrition; noncommunicable diseases; tuberculosis; malaria; and so on (requirement depends on scope of health topics)
- Medical specialty departments: dermatology, mental health, and so on (required for telemedicine; optional for health hotline)
- Health regulatory bodies (Medical or Nurses Council)
- Ministry of Finance (needed for initial establishment, strategic plans, and sustainability planning)
- Ministry of Justice (needed for initial establishment, strategic plans, and sustainability planning)
- Ministry of Communication (communications regulatory bodies)
- All major MNOs that would be linked to the services
- Relevant donors
- Service providers
- National Health Sciences Research Committee (not in stakeholders list but may be relevant)
- Representatives of academic and research institutions (not in stakeholders list but may be relevant)
- Other relevant partners
- Other specialized organizations (may be called in as the need for their expertise arises)

Note: The planning task force has its own terms of reference.

Subcommittee (Telemedicine or Health Hotline Policy Development Regulatory Subcommittee)

Purpose: The purpose of the subcommittee is to prepare, plan, and coordinate policy and regulatory guidelines related to telemedicine or health hotlines. The subcommittee will also share lessons with the main committee.

Responsibilities

- Develop policy for [select: national telemedicine or hotline] services.
- Monitor policy and regulatory adherence to [select: national telemedicine or hotline] services.
- Share resources from other countries.
- Report to the full steering committee on any specific tasks.

Membership

The subcommittee will be led by the Ministry of Health Department of Policy and Planning and include the following:

- Ministry of Justice
- Ministry of Health (whichever department stewards the [select: national telemedicine or hotline] services)
- Health regulatory bodies (Nurses and Medical Council)
- Ministry of Communications regulatory body
- Others as needed

ANNEX 5B. TELEMEDICINE OR HEALTH HOTLINE FIVE-YEAR STRATEGY DECISION-MAKING TOOL

Purpose: The Telemedicine or Health Hotline Five-Year Strategy Decision-Making Tool provides the questions that the government must answer to align its vision around the following aspects of the service:

- Solution management
- Solution impact or outcome
- Health area
- Services
- Geographic coverage

Timing: The steering committee should develop the initial five-year strategy after the planning task force has completed the high-level solution design and the steering committee has validated the design. The five-year strategy will be iterative, because it may require revamping once costing is possible.

Instructions: Before the steering committee meeting, the focal point and planning task force should individually get input from members of the steering committee and present the background information at the steering committee meeting. The focal point with the planning task force can help facilitate a discussion at a steering committee meeting to help further develop and validate this five-year strategy. The focal point should guide the discussion to ensure the steering committee comes to a consensus on the overall vision of the services.

The strategy is the basis for all other planning. Without a solid strategy, it will be difficult to build out a request for proposal from service providers or to budget a five-year plan. Establishing even the solution management vision by year will help all stakeholders (government, service providers, donors, and so on) align on the pathway to sustainability from the outset.

	QUESTIONS TO ANSWER IN EACH YEAR	1	2	3	4	5
Solution coverage summary of table						
Note: Insert answers from the areas below	*Reach [insert number] of [clients: insert health worker or direct community user] for [insert health areas] by providing [insert all that apply: telemedicine, hotline, interactive voice recording, Short Message Service, and so forth] in [insert geographic coverage] led by [insert government or service provider] to improve [insert outcome or impact indicator] by [x] percent.*					
Solution management	*In this year, who will lead the service? [Answer: government, service provider, or co-led]*					
Solution outcome or impact	*What outcome or impact would you like to achieve this year? (Note: Outcome indicators will likely be used for the first two years and the government or partner and donor should plan for an impact evaluation after two years.)*					
Health areas	List health areas (one area per row) — *How many clients do you hope to reach in this health area through the service?*					
	[Example] Maternal and child health					
	xxx					
Services	Hotline — *For this service, list what health area you will offer in this year. List not applicable if you will not offer it.*					
	Voice messages					
	Short Message Service					
	WhatsApp					
	xxx					
Geographic coverage	List health area by geographic coverage — *[Insert health area] in [number of districts, provinces, counties, and so on]. List specific names if known.*					

ANNEX 5C. SAMPLE TELEMEDICINE OR HEALTH HOTLINE FIVE-YEAR STRATEGY

Background: This Sample Telemedicine or Health Hotline Five-Year Strategy (https://thedocs.worldbank.org/en/doc/320f69950dbd48cfb32d6d25ad9b30ca -0390012023/original/5C-Government-Toolkit-Example-Telemedicine-Health -Hotline-5-year-Strategy.pptx) shows the projection a government may take. Years 1 and 2 are filled as examples.

	YEAR 1	YEAR 2	YEAR 3	YEAR 4	YEAR 5
Solution coverage summary of table	*Reach 50,000 clients for MNCH by providing hotline and voice message services in two provinces led by a social enterprise in order to improve access time with health personnel by 67 percent*	*Reach 130,000 clients for MNCH and SRH by providing hotline and voice message services (and WhatsApp for MNCH) in four provinces led by a social enterprise in order to increase likelihood of having children under two vaccinated by 20 percent*	…	…	…
Solution management	*Social enterprise–led*	*Social enterprise–led*	*Co-led*	*Co-led*	*Government-led*
Solution outcome or impact	*Time with health personnel increased from 3 minutes (in facility) to 5 minutes (hotline)*	*Increased likelihood of having children under two vaccinated from 75 to 95 percent*	…	…	…
Health areas	MNCH	50,000 clients	70,000 clients	…	…	…
	SRH	*n.a.*	60,000 clients	…	…	…
	All health topics	*n.a.*	*n.a.*	…	…	…
Services	Hotline	MNCH	MNCH, SRH	…	…	…
	Voice messages	MNCH	MNCH, SRH	…	…	…
	SMS	*n.a.*	*n.a.*	…	…	…
	WhatsApp	*n.a.*	MNCH	…	…	…
	XXX	*n.a.*	*n.a.*	…	…	…
Geographic coverage	*MNCH: Province 1, 2*	*MNCH, SRH: Province 1, 2, 3, 4*	…	…	…

Note: MNCH = maternal, newborn, and child health; n.a. = not applicable; SMS = Short Message Service; SRH = sexual and reproductive health.

NOTE

1. The Malawi Ministry of Health used a dedicated steering committee; however, other governments may choose to use existing forums that already pull from the majority of needed decision-makers. Those governments would then invite the additional organizations and ministries needed for that particular validation meeting (such as a senior management meeting or a relevant technical working group). The key is that the body has the authority to make decisions and sign off on the strategic plans, road maps, budget, and so on. Although ministers of health usually do the final sign-off, prior agreement by their directors is a way of formalizing the decision.

Plan to Engage with the Private Sector

Now that the government understands what it wants to achieve with the five-year strategy, it needs to consider how to engage the private sector service providers. It is important to complete the private sector strategy before completing the one-year road map or choosing service providers, because the strategy will determine which activities the work plan needs to include and will define the nature of private sector involvement in the solution. Chapter 6 helps governments create a private sector strategy and understand how to engage with mobile network operators. It presents the following tool and reference materials:

- *Private Sector Strategy Worksheet (annex 6A)*
- *Understanding Types of Collaboration with the Private Sector Reference Materials (annex 6B)*

DEVELOP A PRIVATE SECTOR STRATEGY

Developing a private sector strategy requires first completing the five-year strategy. As part of developing the five-year strategy, the government made key decisions on which elements to operate internally (using government employees and infrastructure) and which to outsource to private sector partners. The steering committee should develop the private sector strategy using the Private Sector Strategy Worksheet in annex 6A.

It is important to involve all key stakeholders in development of the private sector strategy. In addition to ministry of health personnel, the government may need to involve other departments, such as the ministry of communications, and possibly external bodies such as trade associations. Key stakeholders include those departments and individuals whose involvement will be needed to execute the private sector strategy.

Whatever the private sector contribution or type of collaboration, the government needs to remain the solution steward and should therefore

- Define the functional requirements;
- Define the performance framework and associated performance targets; and
- Assess performance and ensure corrective actions are in place if the solution does not provide the targeted impact.

If a government private sector strategy requires using types of collaboration for which the government has little experience, it is important that the government include private sector collaboration capacity-building activities during the first year.

For more information on collaborations, see the Understanding Types of Collaboration with the Private Sector Reference Materials in annex 6B.

BEGIN STRATEGIC CONVERSATIONS WITH MOBILE NETWORK OPERATORS TO ZERO-RATE CALLS AND ESTABLISH SHORT CODES

Despite the importance in low- and middle-income countries of providing services free to the public, some governments in those countries cannot take on the cost of calls made for health services. Governments will therefore need mobile network operators (MNOs) to establish zero-rate calls. If the government has not already engaged MNOs in strategic conversations regarding the potential to zero-rate calls and Short Message Service (SMS), if needed, and to establish short codes, it should start immediately.[1] The government should decide whether to engage all MNOs in the country or if select MNOs could cover the country fully. In some countries, a leading MNO has wide enough coverage; in others, ensuring coverage across the country might require two or more MNOs.

Although MNOs should already have participated in the steering committee, it often takes constant and persistent contact with them before they engage with the government. In addition to using the private sector strategy to develop a partnership with an MNO, the government should also

- Highlight the mutual benefit, such as appealing to the corporate social responsibility department and the elevation of the MNO's service offering;
- Understand that the MNO may have an exclusivity clause[2] and decide how to handle it depending on the country context;
- Set up regular check-ins and make a written plan to work toward short codes and zero-rating;
- Understand the MNO's approval cycles; and
- Use the highest-level contacts (ministers of health, secretaries for health, and so on) to speak to the MNO's managing director or highest official.

Once the government has an agreement with an MNO, it should develop a memorandum of understanding (Phase 3) to ensure mutual understanding of roles. (Note: Because they are critical to establishing and sustaining the services, conversations with MNOs need to happen sooner than similar conversations with technology service providers when contracts are in place—Phase 4.)

ANNEX 6A. PRIVATE SECTOR STRATEGY WORKSHEET

Purpose: The Private Sector Strategy Worksheet assists governments in documenting a private sector strategy for a given solution such as a health hotline service. By filling out the worksheet, governments will have a simple, usable private sector strategy. In addition to the strategy, the government will need action plans, which are not included in the worksheet.

Timing: The Private Sector Strategy Worksheet can be completed at the same time as the five-year strategy or afterward. Because the two strategies are likely to be iterative, parallel development is recommended.

Instructions:
1. *Purpose of this document:* This section is prefilled and provides guidance on the purpose of the strategy and the types of collaboration included. It also provides a reminder that the strategy is not designed to support management of specific relationships. You will need to add the name of the solution that is the focus of the private sector strategy.
2. *Objectives:* Use this section to specify the objectives, scope (product and geography), stage (targeting, contracting, partnering), outcomes expected, and start and end dates of the collaboration. Each specific outcome should have its own dedicated line.
3. *Key principles:* Use this section to document the principles that govern any collaboration with the private sector. Principles typically address topics such as competition and exclusivity, key minimum requirements, unbundling of product and service provision, and adherence to government-defined standards. The following examples could apply to a telemedicine or health hotline service:
   - "We support equal access to the service for all clients, so we aim for partnerships with mobile service providers that enable equal access."
   - "Telecom partners that take the risk of early involvement should be rewarded with exclusivity for a period not exceeding three years."
   - "Partners are required to adhere to the approved solution standard operating procedures and contribute to ongoing updates of these procedures."
   - "Partners must commit to implementing practices that respect standards related to client confidentiality."
   - "Partners must commit to implementing practices that ensure network security to protect data and avoid fraudulent use of the service."
4. *Strategy review:* Use this section to indicate the frequency at which this strategy needs to be reviewed and updated.
5. *Approvals:* Use this section to record the signatures of stakeholders key to the strategy.

PRIVATE SECTOR STRATEGY	**Program name:** *xxx*

1. Purpose of this document

This document describes the needed contributions from the private sector for the *xxx* program and sets out objectives, principles, and dates that will guide the targeting of, recruiting of, contracting of, and partnering with private sector partners. All private sector contributions are in scope and include financial and service donations, technical assistance, product provision, and service provision. Despite possible opportunities for synergies across programs, this strategy is specific to the *xxx* program.

This document does not focus on a given private sector partner and is therefore not suitable for managing a specific private sector partner relationship. Such a relationship will require specific contracts, memorandums of understanding, and service-level agreements.

2. Objectives: List the objectives, scope (product and geography), stage (targeting, contracting, partnering), names of partners, outcomes expected, and collaboration start and end dates.

Add general observations on the role of public-private engagement in this solution.

Objectives	Scope	Stage	Partner/potential partners	Targeted outcomes	Collaboration start and end

3. Key principles: List the key principles that must be applied to all private sector partners.

a)   *xxx*

b)   *xxx*

4. Strategy review: **Indicate date or frequency for review of this strategy.**

This strategy should be reviewed every *x* months.

5. Approvals

ANNEX 6B. UNDERSTANDING TYPES OF COLLABORATION WITH THE PRIVATE SECTOR REFERENCE MATERIALS

To gain the benefits of working with the private sector requires mastering collaboration. The government can engage the private sector as part of a health solution in many ways, including but not limited to the following:

- Purchasing software or equipment for a call center
- Contracting for provision and maintenance of all or some needed hardware and software
- Contracting a private call center to set up and run the telemedicine or health hotline services
- Obtaining free or subsidized communications and promotion of telemedicine or hotline services in exchange for allowing the MNO to achieve its corporate social responsibility or marketing objectives

The different engagements with the private sector in turn require specific types of collaboration. In this case, collaboration is defined as working toward mutual objectives through the sharing of ideas, assets, information, knowledge, risks, and rewards. Collaborative relationships can deliver major benefits to both the government and its private sector partners. For example, in Malawi, as part of its corporate and social responsibility branch, Airtel agreed to zero-rate the calls for Chipatala Cha Pa Foni, or Health Center by Phone. Community member interest in using the service in one district led to requests for additional cell towers and the expansion of Airtel's business within that district.

The government's experience with private sector collaboration will dictate the activities necessary for a successful partnership. For example, governments with low levels of experience may need to implement specific capacity-building activities to engage productively with the private sector. The Collaboration Model Guidance shown in table 6B.1 provides an overview of three types of collaboration with the private sector.

1. *Transactional collaboration* is used when the opportunity is limited to increasing the efficiency of interactions, such as simplifying ordering and receiving.
2. *Cooperative collaboration* is useful when jointly defined processes are needed for each partner to achieve its performance targets—typically the case when the service provider is providing an important component of the solution, such as information technology maintenance.
3. *Coordinated collaboration* is typically used when jointly defined targets and action plans for cost, service, and quality are essential—typically the case when the service provider is responsible for managing or operating part of the solution.

Each type has varying levels of investments and benefits. Depending on the full scope of the solution, a government may have several transactional collaborations, fewer cooperative collaborations, and very few, or only one, coordinated collaborations. Governments generally have few of the last type because of the high level of investment required for relationship management and codevelopment of processes and tools.

It is important to understand the difference between the three types of collaboration and how they apply to different ways of engaging with the private sector. For example, applying a transactional collaboration model with a private sector firm operating a call center on behalf of a government will likely result in a less effective collaboration because of missing key management practices.

TABLE 6B.1 Collaboration model guidance

	TRANSACTIONAL	COOPERATIVE	COORDINATED
Examples	Private sector supplies software or equipment for a call center.	Mobile network operator provides zero-rated or subsidized calls in exchange for marketing visibility. Private sector provides and maintains all needed hardware and software.	Private call center sets up and runs services.
Needed collaborative practices	Share project plans with contracted suppliers to inform suppliers' planning. Share supply plans with government customer to inform call center plans.	Transactional practices: • Service-level agreements • Jointly defined standard operating procedures • Shared access to information systems or systems integration protocols	Transactional and cooperative practices: • Joint sharing of benefits and savings • Joint business planning
Examples of benefits	Government: Items are available at a competitive price on time. Private sector: Able to forward plan production or service provision and avoid costs of expediting.	Government: Service meets government requirements and provides benefits of private sector experience and costs. Private sector: Collaboration with government through agreed processes and procedures can enable greater efficiencies.	Government: Collaboration results in ongoing service and cost improvement. Private sector: Collaboration creates potential for greater profitability through gainsharing agreements.
Potential disadvantages	None	Requires investments in shared standard operating procedures; very difficult to implement if a quality management system is not in place.	Requires a high level of relationship management; will not work if individuals don't have collaboration skills.

If a government private sector strategy requires using types of collaboration for which the government has little experience, it is important that the government include private sector collaboration capacity-building activities as part of its Year 1 plan.

NOTES

1. *Zero-rating calls* means that the MNO provides all incoming calls (and outgoing calls and SMS, if negotiated) free to the government (or whoever runs the service on behalf of the government). Because the cost of SMS is often much higher, MNOs are not always willing to zero-rate these messages; however, it is worth negotiating if the government thinks SMS is critical to the overall services. *Short codes* are the numbers generally used for services rather than long individual numbers and are often provided at a reduced price or zero-rated. For example, in the United State, 911 is used for emergency services because it is quick and free to the caller.

2. An *exclusivity clause* in this context is when an MNO requires that the short code be used or zero-rated only for users of its network and not for other mobile network providers in the country.

Plan to Have a Working System within a Year

Chapter 7 builds upon the five-year strategy and private sector strategy to help governments develop a one-year road map for getting the system up and running. It presents the following tool and reference materials:

- Editable One-Year Road Map (annex 7A)
- Understanding Project Personnel Needed Reference Materials (annex 7B)

DEVELOP A ONE-YEAR ROAD MAP

Once the government has a vision of what it hopes the solution will achieve, it should plan the major milestones and tasks that require partner input for the first year. A telemedicine or health hotline service can be planned, operating, and functional within a year—or even within three months, if the government chooses the outsourced solution option. The one-year road map in figure 7.1 includes the activities for Phases 0–4; however, for the purposes of this toolkit, the government should review Phases 0–2.[1] The one-year road map assumes that the government has chosen to outsource the solution initially.[2] As part of starting up/operationalizing, the road map should include base actions required to ensure sustainability, as outlined in the five-year strategy. Actions for sustainability need to be built into the design. If a government wants services that later operate within the ministry of health (in-house option), it will need to identify a building or build a new structure, which could take time.[3] The one-year road map can be adapted as needed for the respective country (see the Editable One-Year Road Map in annex 7A). For more information on the telemedicine or health hotline management and implementation personnel needed to actualize the one-year road map, see the Understanding Project Personnel Needed Reference Materials in annex 7B.

FIGURE 7.1

One-year road map for telemedicine or health hotline planning and establishment

Activities by phase	1	2	3	4	5	6	7	8	9	10	11	12	Year 2 – 1
Phase 0: Assess basic requirements and express interest	▲												
Determine that country meets basic political stability and technical considerations	▲												
Phase 1: Scope and design solution													
Establish focal point and planning task force	█												
Conduct predesign scoping for health area and target audience	█												
Conduct landscape analysis of in-country service providers	█	█											
Complete initial high-level functional design draft of telemedicine or health hotline services		▲											
Phase 2: Develop strategy, implementation road map, and budget													
Establish cross-sectoral decision-making steering committee			▲										
Validate initial functional and technical design with steering committee			█										
Develop five-year strategy (including sustainability plan)			█	█									
Develop private sector strategy			█										
Begin conversations with MNOs on potential to zero-rate calls and establish short codes			█	█									
Develop one-year road map			█	█									
Release RFQ to get costing and preliminarily select service provider partners			▲										
Cost five-year strategy and one-year road map according to RFP budgets			█	█									
Validate five-year strategy, one-year road map, and budget			▲										
Phase 3ᵃ: Secure funding for startup													
Secure start-up funding					▲								
Establish MOU with MNO to zero-rate calls and establish short codes					▲								
Phase 4: Establish and implement solutionᵇ													
Hold steering committee meetings quarterly					▲		▲		▲		▲		▲
Finalize technical design and contract					█	█							
Build additional content and validate with government					█	█	█						
Begin user testing with refined design testing					█	█	█						
Train hotline workers on new scope or telemedicine practitioners on the platform					█	█							
Advertise service							█	█	█	█	█	█	█
Implement							█	█	█	█	█	█	█

Source: VillageReach.
Note: MNO = mobile network operator; MOU = memorandum of understanding; RFP = request for proposal; RFQ = request for quotation.
a. This road map assumes funding has been identified. Phase 3 milestones include only MNO-related activities. This road map jumps from Phase 2 to Phase 4. Phase 3 funding can take a long and unspecified amount of time.
b. Phase 4 includes establishing, implementing, scaling, and sustaining; however, scaling and sustaining are not in the scope of the one-year road map. The five-year strategy does include sustainability planning.

ANNEX 7A. EDITABLE ONE-YEAR ROAD MAP

Purpose: The purpose of the Editable One-Year Road Map (https://thedocs .worldbank.org/en/doc/e1d2a0943a4f15812edc462215707f98-0390012023 /original/7A-Editable-One-Year-Roadmap-for-Telemedicine-Health-Hotline .pptx) is to help governments plan out major milestones and tasks that they, and their chosen partners, plan to accomplish in the first year of solution planning, setup, and implementation in line with the five-year strategy.

Timing: The planning task force should complete this road map after the steering committee has developed the five-year strategy and private sector strategy.

Instructions: The planning task force should get individual inputs from members of the steering committee to understand the parameters affecting timing for planning and implementation. Ideally, the planning task force would then meet as a group to align on the activities by phase and timing for each milestone or set of activities.

Activities by phase	Year 1												Year 2
	1	2	3	4	5	6	7	8	9	10	11	12	1
Phase 0: Assess basic requirements and express interest	▲												
Determine that country meets basic political stability and technical considerations	▲												
Phase 1: Scope and design solution													
Establish focal point and planning task force	▰												
Conduct predesign scoping for health area and target audience	▰												
Conduct landscape analysis of in-country service providers	▰												
Complete initial high-level functional design draft of telemedicine or health hotline services			▲										
Phase 2: Develop strategy, implementation road map, and budget													
Establish cross-sectoral decision-making steering committee			▲										
Validate initial functional and technical design with steering committee			▲										
Develop five-year strategy (including sustainability plan)			▰										
Develop private sector strategy			▰										
Begin conversations with mobile network operators on potential to zero-rate calls and establish short codes			▰										
Develop one-year road map			▰										
Release request for quotation to get costing and preliminarily select service provider partners			▲										
Cost five-year strategy and one-year road map according to request for proposal budgets			▰										
Validate five-year strategy, one-year road map, and budget			▲										
Phase 3: Secure funding for startup													
Secure start-up funding			▲										
Establish memorandum of understanding with mobile network operator to zero-rate calls and establish short codes			▲										
Phase 4: Establish and implement solution													
Hold steering committee meetings quarterly			▲			▲			▲			▲	
Finalize technical design and contract					▰								
Build additional content and validate with government					▰								
Begin user testing with refined design testing					▰								
Train hotline workers on new scope or telemedicine practitioners on the platform					▰								
Advertise service						▰▰▰▰▰▰▰▰							
Implement						▰▰▰▰▰▰▰▰							

ANNEX 7B. UNDERSTANDING PROJECT PERSONNEL NEEDED REFERENCE MATERIALS

To complete the one-year road map and understand associated costs, the government should understand the personnel needed, starting in Phase 4, to operate the solution. The one-year road map process requires that the government understand the project structure needed to manage and establish the telemedicine or health hotline services in Phase 4. Figure 7B.1 shows the personnel structures needed from both the government and the service provider sides in an outsourced personnel structure model. The telemedicine physicians or health hotline workers may move from the service provider to a government team if the government decides to start with an outsourced solution model and move toward an in-house solution model.

Whether the government chooses the outsourced or in-house solution model in the short or long term, the solution needs dedicated government personnel to oversee its establishment and initial implementation. Because the service provider team in figure 7B.1 includes the existing experts on implementing the solution, this team is critical to ensuring solution quality while establishing or expanding the service to meet the government needs set out in the five-year strategy and one-year road map. If the government will eventually operate and not just outsource services, the service provider team is responsible for transferring its skills to the government. On the government side, it is important to establish the following roles:

- Manager of service provider's implementation and transfer (if applicable)
- Key decision-making focal point within the government (usually the head of the department that stewards the telemedicine or hotline services)
- Focal point for monitoring and evaluation at the ministry to ensure the government has data for decision-making
- Technical experts (both health area and information technology) to ensure the content used is revised, validated, and used appropriately

FIGURE 7B.1

Telemedicine or health hotline management and implementation personnel

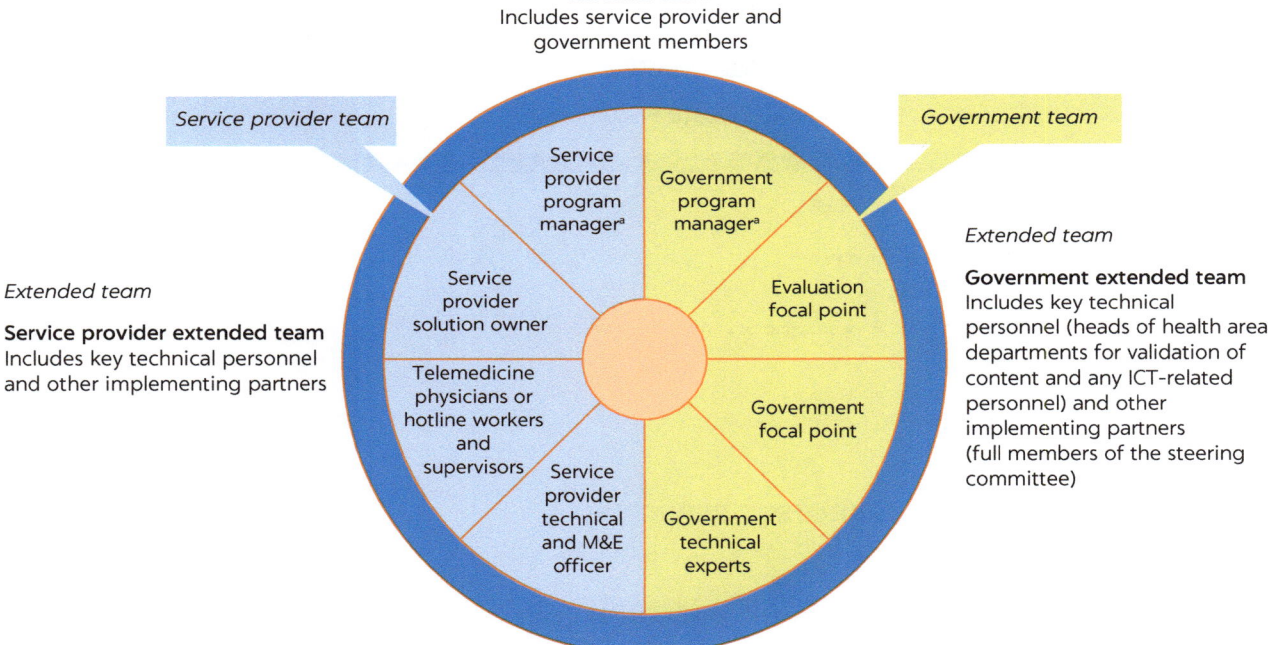

Source: Original figure developed for this publication.
Note: ICT = information and communication technology; M&E = monitoring and evaluation.
a. The service provider program manager and government program manager for the telemedicine or hotline services drive the establishment and ongoing implementation.

NOTES

1. Figure 7.1 also gives precursory milestones for what would happen in Phase 4 within one year, assuming Phase 3 funding has been identified. It is not actually possible, however, to move forward with Phase 4 without funding, or if funding for the solution was not already allocated through government funding cycles, which usually take place yearly. Donor funding may also take a long time. During COVID-19, many governments and partners received quick funding for pandemic-related purposes that could be leveraged for quick setup; but the ability to set up quickly depends greatly on the government's ability to validate scope, design, and content quickly.

2. If the government manages the solution in-house and then outsources, it will waste resources; however, outsourcing first then managing in-house or managing in-house throughout (with some outsourced components as needed) is acceptable.

3. In Malawi, Chipatala Cha Pa Foni, or Health Center by Phone, operated from the district hospital, even when originally operated by VillageReach. When scaling up, the Ministry of Health identified a building on its national capital Health Education Unit grounds, which reduced the cost of building a new structure and made the transfer to full government ownership easier.

## 8

Select the Best Technologies and Partners for a Sustainable Integrated Solution

Once the government has completed all the previous tools and steps, it is time to select preliminary technologies and partners to cost the five-year strategy and one-year road map. Chapter 8 helps the government understand what types of technologies and partners to look for in preparing a request for proposal or quotation, how to develop the terms of reference for such requests, the pros and cons of using existing services, major technical considerations, how to ensure compliance with regulatory bodies from the outset, how to position telemedicine or health hotline services within national health information system architectures and health information exchanges, how to develop a national plan for aligning and governing multiple telemedicine or health hotline services, and how to begin long-term strategic conversations with mobile network operators. Understanding each of these activities will help the government set up for success and develop a costing for the five-year strategy and one-year road map. Chapter 8 presents the following tools:

- *Overall Technical Considerations Checklist (annex 8A)*
- *Government's Telemedicine or Health Hotline Services Terms of Reference Development Checklist (annex 8B)*
- *Selection Criteria Matrix (annex 8C)*

SELECT PARTNERS TO FILL EXISTING GAPS TO EXPAND REACH OF HEALTH CARE SYSTEM

When selecting technologies or partners to expand the reach of the health care system, begin by clearly articulating the previously identified needs and priorities for the service. Generally, it is best to progressively develop the partnership with a smaller scope of work and learn from that experience. Although the aim of this toolkit is to help governments plan for nationwide services, there are ways to create a phased approach either by geography or by health areas. Additionally, if the partner has a proven solution, the service would build upon what that partner already has.

From the start, make sure to select a service provider using a competitive procurement process led by the government. To ensure selection of the best technology or partner, be organized and clear about the goals of the procurement process.

Best practices for selecting the technology or partner include the following:

- Having a selection committee that includes technical and nontechnical representatives
- Viewing demonstrations of the services
- Interviewing prior users or customers of the service to understand their experience
- Carefully evaluating costs and features
- Using a scoring rubric to help evaluate and select the best platform

Consider a partner or technology platform with services in the country and with existing government relationships. Partners that already understand a country's existing e-strategy, integration strategies, and needs often provide the best fit. One component of a country's policy that is particularly helpful to know and consider is its existing regulations for storing data (that is, requirements for cloud-based versus in-country hosting versus external servers).

For health hotline implementations specifically, consider an outsourced solution partner that has a plan for anticipated call volumes and the ability to determine what staffing or services will be needed to reach a high call answer rate with low wait times. Additionally, to manage the demand as service usage grows, consider service providers that can integrate alternative methods of meeting demand that use artificial intelligence or prerecorded messages (such as interactive voice response or chatbot), because having high numbers of hotline workers and staff can become financially unsustainable for the government.

UNDERSTAND THE MAJOR TECHNICAL CONSIDERATIONS

The major technical considerations when building or selecting a service provider for telemedicine or health hotline services are connectivity, systems and software development, maintenance, data storage, safety and privacy, hardware installation and maintenance, and human resource training. Although the minimum technical considerations were already discussed in chapter 2 and laid out in the Minimum Technical Considerations Checklist (annex 2B), this section provides more details to scope beyond the basic technical requirements. The following information is the basis for the Overall Technical Considerations Checklist in annex 8A.

Connectivity

For both telemedicine and health hotlines to operate, they need reliable internet connectivity. Factors to consider for connectivity are coverage, quality, and cost. A health hotline needs the internet primarily on the operational side to run the servers and hotline services. The client side requires cellular access (but not internet data) because the interaction is voice-based and runs through mobile networks. Hotlines that provide additional services by Short Message Service, Unstructured Supplementary Service Data, WhatsApp, or social messaging will require data bundling and additional funding to operate the service. Unlike a health hotline, telemedicine requires reliable internet connection on both ends, the operational side (doctor or hospital) and the patient side. The quality of the internet connection also matters, because telemedicine requires access to a good broadband internet connection, the cost of which varies from country to country.[1] Carefully consider the solution's target population, because internet connectivity also varies greatly by location.

Ensure systems and software development, upgrade, and maintenance

Telemedicine or health hotline services require scalable software systems to handle caller demand that varies over time. System scalability is "a measure of a system's ability to increase or decrease in performance and cost in response to changes in application and system processing demands."[2] Software platforms should be user-friendly and should, ideally, require zero to minimal software developer intervention to change content over time to meet a country's health system gaps. Make sure to identify one-time and recurring costs—including any software license costs, feature upgrade costs, and ongoing maintenance. Scalable systems also ensure the affordability and ease of adding features and upgrading capacity.

Provide data storage safety and privacy

Health data storage and hosting services represent a sensitive topic that needs careful consideration. In many countries, the government requires in-country storage of health data, which may make it possible to use private data centers (in-country) as well as public or government data centers. In either case, the government should identify how it will manage hosting and storing data. Table 8.1 provides details on the characteristics of governments' options:

- Cloud data- or systems-hosting services (fee-based subscription or pay-as-you-go)
- On-premises server-hosting facilities (purchasing and managing server hardware)

Ensure data protection and appropriate data sharing

Ensuring the privacy of health information requires carefully implementing data safety and privacy measures. This process begins with securing end-to-end connectivity used in transmission, servers, and workstations, as well as physical facility security. Additionally, service provider policies will need to be in place to ensure that caller information remains confidential.

The government should follow the country's existing e-strategy, digital health, or monitoring and evaluation data protection and data-sharing policies and best practices. Table 8.2 lays out key areas for the government to consider, all of which may affect data protection.

It is critical that governments work with all partners to establish a data-sharing agreement that includes how to store data in accordance with the country's standards. Governments will often want to own the data; however, if all or some of the elements of the service are operated by a service provider or funder, that stakeholder would likely need access to data for service delivery and for data dashboards. The government should provide clear guidance on (1) who should

TABLE 8.1 Overview of data storage and hosting services characteristics

	CLOUD SERVICES	ON PREMISES
Resilience and elasticity	Downtime almost zero, with flexible space and capacity	Not as flexible; limited capacity and computing power
Flexibility and scalability	Easy and low-cost scaling	Needs additional resources, making it costly to change
Running costs	No additional costs for hardware and support service	Additional hardware and support services costs
	Higher running cost of the internet because everything needs internet connection to access	Low internet cost because systems can be accessed through the local network
	Reduced power cost because most computing power hardware is outsourced	Potentially higher cost of power to run hardware
Security	Potentially less secure at times because data privacy and security depend on the provider	Allows owner to control data privacy and security
	Guaranteed data availability	Potentially less-assured data availability because it depends on effectiveness of the infrastructure implementation

Source: LeadingEdge, "How Is Cloud Computing Different from Traditional IT Infrastructure?" (https://www.leadingedgetech.co.uk/it-services/it-consultancy-services/cloud-computing/how-is-cloud-computing-different-from-traditional-it-infrastructure/).

TABLE 8.2 Key areas that affect data protection

AREA	CONSIDERATIONS
Staff policies	Confidentiality agreements and other policies about getting support from supervisors or other colleagues while on calls or telemedicine videos
Physical equipment	Where the equipment is, who has access to it, and what needs to be done to limit access
Facility	Where the facility is located, who has access to it, and what needs to be done to limit access
Protocols	• Outline how to achieve safe storage, who can access information, and what information can be shared • Label which variables or sets of variables are identifiers • Describe how data can be shared between different stakeholders • Identify what can and cannot be analyzed according to the confidentiality agreements
Patient privacy	Confidentiality agreements, storage of recordings and videos, and identifying who has access

Source: Original table developed for this publication.

have access to the raw data, (2) who can have access to the aggregated data, and (3) who is responsible for aggregating the data. When selecting a service provider partner, the government should be clear about data-sharing expectations from the beginning.

Ensure cybersecurity

Cybersecurity is "the practice of protecting systems, networks, and programs from digital attacks."[3] These cyberattacks (https://www.cisco.com/c/en/us/products/security/common-cyberattacks.html) usually aim at "accessing, changing, or destroying sensitive information; extorting money from users via ransomware; or interrupting normal business processes." Data breaches—which cause enormous loss and tarnish companies' reputations, often resulting in lawsuits—have become notorious across the media in the past few years. Cyberattacks in telemedicine or health hotline services typically involve gaining access to communication networks and listening in on conversations, gaining access to patients' private information, or gaining access to communication servers and systems to steal airtime or make malicious, expensive calls. Numerous laws and regulations, both international and country-specific, deal with cybersecurity. For instance, Malawi's Electronic Transactions and Cyber Security Act of 2016 prohibits and imposes heavy fines on unauthorized access to, interception of, or interference with data and computer systems.[4]

Because these laws and regulations can be executed only after a digital attack, prevention matters. Mobile network operators, and any other service providers, must clearly articulate who has the responsibility for setting up any protective security measures in the system. Doing so will help avoid blame and strained relationships if cyberattacks occur. Cybersecurity measures include the use of firewalls, antivirus software, intrusion detection and prevention systems, encryption, and login passwords to systems and devices. Also important are ongoing training and reinforcement with staff about security and privacy expectations, including how to identify and report suspect activity.

Hardware installation and maintenance

In the case of an in-house solution model, telemedicine or health hotline services will require the acquisition of hardware such as workstation computers, phones, computer networks (wired or wireless), power backup systems, servers, solar power, battery backups, and more. Make sure to plan for up-front (one-time) purchase costs for necessary hardware, as well as for ongoing maintenance, upgrades, and periodic replacement. The type of hardware needed will depend on whether the government wants to own and operate the hardware or to contract with a service provider. For ongoing hardware support, the government can either allocate dedicated staff or subcontract with an information technology support contractor. This decision will depend on the size and complexity of the chosen hardware. Table 8.3 shows the pros and cons of having dedicated staff versus having a contractor.

Human resource training

No service will succeed without well-trained staff to operate it. The early stages of solution development need to involve any staff who will be providing supporting services or working with any software or hardware (that is, during systems

TABLE 8.3 Pros and cons of staffing information technology support (in-house solution model)

	ARRANGEMENT	COST IMPLICATION	EFFECTIVENESS
Dedicated staff	**Always on site**	High cost because staff are paid regardless of workload	High efficiency because staff are always available to respond to issues as they happen
Information technology support contractor	**On-call billing**	Low cost because contractor bills per hour spent on an issue	• Potential delay in contractor's response to an issue • Potential for contractor to spend more time resolving an issue to increase billing hours
	Monthly billing	• Better for budgeting because it can be combined with other monthly bills • Constant billing regardless of increase or decrease of workload • Potentially higher cost than hiring dedicated staff, assuming in both cases one staff member assigned to duty station	Effective, assuming the contractor's presence on site to respond to any issue at any time (often includes predetermined work hours or response guarantees)

Source: Original table developed for this publication.

development, hardware installations). Whether in-house or outsourced, staff members need training not only on health topics but also on software and hardware use. Any company offering telemedicine or health hotline services to the government should share information on how the company trains, assesses, and retains its staff. If the government will take on the service, it is important that all related government personnel are also trained to operate the service.

POSITION TELEMEDICINE OR HEALTH HOTLINE SERVICES WITHIN NATIONAL HEALTH INFORMATION SYSTEM ARCHITECTURES AND HEALTH INFORMATION EXCHANGES

As with data protection, it is critical that the government-stewarded solution follow any e-health governance and decision-making structures. Although not all countries have national electronic medical records, governments working toward that capacity would want to ensure these services could become interoperable for future health information exchanges. Ensuring the interoperability of any telemedicine or hotline services will give the government the option to display different services on one dashboard. It will also be helpful when connecting clients with health centers or emergency transport when referred. Because many governments are in the process of simultaneously rolling out new services, it will be critical for the solution focal point to actively participate in any e-health governance technical working groups, along with any chosen service providers for a telemedicine or hotline service, to understand the required interoperability.

In being interoperable and part of the national architecture, it is advisable to use open standards—for example, HL7 International's FHIR[5] for communication standards and SNOMED, ICD, and LOINC among others for clinical content.[6] Additionally, the OpenHIE Community is a great resource for learning more about interoperability.[7]

DEVELOP REQUEST FOR PROPOSAL OR QUOTATION WITH TERMS OF REFERENCE FOR SERVICE PROVIDERS

Once it has taken into account the solution design, five-year strategy, one-year road map, and all the private sector and technical considerations, the government will be ready to establish terms of reference (TOR) to solicit a request for proposal (RFP) or a request for quotation (RFQ) from service providers.

An RFP or RFQ typically contains four major components:

1. List of required documentation from the vendor (company background, experience and financial information, compliance-related information, and so on)
2. TOR document that provides a description of the government's requirements to the vendor
3. Required points the vendor must cover in its response to the government's TOR, including a work plan
4. Quotation or fee schedule template, which the vendor will complete with information on costing and level of effort

Of all these components, the TOR is the most critical because it reflects the government's requirements and their relative importance. Each TOR has unique content that reflects service area specificities, as seen in the Government's Telemedicine or Health Hotline Services Terms of Reference Development Checklist in annex 8B. The checklist includes key areas that typically need to be covered for a telemedicine or health hotline RFP or RFQ. The Selection Criteria Matrix in annex 8C helps governments understand what to look for or consider when selecting a partner.

ANNEX 8A. OVERALL TECHNICAL CONSIDERATIONS CHECKLIST

Purpose: The Overall Technical Considerations Checklist helps governments really understand what technological factors the solution requires and what to consider.

Timing: The government should review the technical considerations checklist when it is ready to explore different potential technology partners.

Instructions: The focal point—or someone in the ministry who understands technology—should fill out the checklist, answering "Yes," "No," or "n.a." (not applicable). This person should then present the information to the planning taskforce and potentially to the steering committee.

#	TECHNICAL AREA	KEY QUESTION/ITEM TO CONSIDER	AVAILABLE?	COMMENT
1	**Connectivity**	**Does the country have good low-cost internet and mobile phone connectivity?**		
	– Coverage	Does the country's population have at least 50 percent broadband internet and 80 percent cell phone coverage?	❏ Yes ❏ No ❏ n.a.	
	– Quality	Is cell phone network uptime at least 90 percent and internet uptime over 80 percent?	❏ Yes ❏ No ❏ n.a.	
	– Cost	Are internet and airtime rates affordable to the average citizen?	❏ Yes ❏ No ❏ n.a.	
2	**Systems and software development upgrade and maintenance**	**Is the service scalable, upgradable, user-friendly, and able to integrate with other systems?**		
	– Scalability	Is the service able to increase or decrease in performance and cost in response to changes in application and system-processing demands?	❏ Yes ❏ No ❏ n.a.	
	– User-friendliness	Are users able to use and make changes to content without the developer's intervention?	❏ Yes ❏ No ❏ n.a.	
	– Upgradability	Is it easy to add system functionalities with minimal time and cost?	❏ Yes ❏ No ❏ n.a.	
	– Integration with other systems	Is the service ready, or can it easily integrate and share data with other systems?	❏ Yes ❏ No ❏ n.a.	

continued

#	TECHNICAL AREA	KEY QUESTION/ITEM TO CONSIDER	AVAILABLE?	COMMENT
3	**Data storage safety and privacy**	**Are data storage, hosting, backup facilities, and data privacy and protection available at all levels?**		
	– Data storage/hosting/ backup facility	Are data storage/hosting/backup available/ accessible in country or cloud based?	❑ Yes ❑ No ❑ n.a.	
	– Staff policies	Are staff confidentiality agreements and other policies available for patient data protection?	❑ Yes ❑ No ❑ n.a.	
	– Physical equipment	Are physical assets, equipment, and facilities physically protected, and are accessibility measures in place?	❑ Yes ❑ No ❑ n.a.	
	– Patient privacy	Are patient confidentiality agreements in place, and is access to storage of recordings and videos controlled and limited?	❑ Yes ❑ No ❑ n.a.	
4	**Hardware installation and maintenance**	**Are you buying your own hardware and support services, or are you renting? If buying, have you planned for maintenance, replacement, or upgrade?**		
	– Purchase of hardware	Are you purchasing hardware, such as workstation computers, phones, computer networks (wired/wireless), power backup systems, servers, solar power, and battery backups?	❑ Yes ❑ No ❑ n.a.	
	– Maintenance	Do you plan to use an in-house support team?	❑ Yes ❑ No ❑ n.a.	
		Are you outsourcing support services?	❑ Yes ❑ No ❑ n.a.	
	– Replacement	Have you budgeted in advance for at least 25 percent hardware replacement within the first three years?	❑ Yes ❑ No ❑ n.a.	
	– Upgrade	Do you plan a software or hardware upgrade in the next five years that will require advance budgeting?	❑ Yes ❑ No ❑ n.a.	
5	**Human resource training**			
	– Technical support staff	Are support staff involved right from systems implementation?	❑ Yes ❑ No ❑ n.a.	
	– Government/hotline personnel	Does the training program include training of trainers for government or hotline staff for sustainability?	❑ Yes ❑ No ❑ n.a.	

ANNEX 8B. GOVERNMENT'S TELEMEDICINE OR HEALTH HOTLINE SERVICES TERMS OF REFERENCE DEVELOPMENT CHECKLIST

Purpose: The Government's Telemedicine or Health Hotline Services Terms of Reference Development Checklist helps governments know what to include in the TOR section of an RFP or RFQ.

Timing: The government will usually release the RFP or RFQ after it has a high-level functional and technical design, a government five-year strategy, and a one-year road map. This RFP or RFQ will include the TOR.

Instructions: Although every government has different contracting templates, the government contract officer can use this checklist as a guideline for what to include as TOR in the RFP or RFQ. The checklist includes the topic, description, and proposed length (in number of pages) of the different TOR elements.

	TOPIC	DESCRIPTION	LENGTH
1.0 Overview			
	Introduction	Present the overall objective of the request for quotation including a view of the overall five-year strategy.	0.5 page
1.1	Background	Explain the history of the need, including scope and key characteristics of any existing solutions; list current performance levels of existing solutions; and list all key locations and assets that will be used.	0.5 page
1.2	Organizations	Explain the key entities and any existing private sector partners that will be involved in implementing and operating the solution.	0.5 page
1.3	Strategy	Describe how this solution fits into overall government strategy.	0.5 page
1.4	Governance	Describe the key stakeholders, champions, and leaders who will provide oversight and decision-making for the request for proposal or request for quotation and the ongoing solution management.	1 page
2.0 Need			
	Introduction	Present the solution scope in terms of health areas, health services, geography, and key targeted health outcomes.	5 pages
2.1	Call center services	List the required services in short sentences with clear sections for outbound calls, inbound calls, and data collection and reporting.	1 page
2.2	Support services	Describe different levels of support for Tier 1, Tier 2, and Tier 3 to specify who should be involved in responding to which requests (call center employees or government staff, and which government staff).	0.5 page
2.3	Service availability	Describe the target availability, reliability, and response times of service described in section 2.1, including a description of normal hours of operations and scheduled downtime.	0.5 page
2.4	Key performance indicators	List the top 4–5 indicators that will be used to measure performance.	0.5 page
2.5	Call volume	Provide the historical and projected call volume.	0.5 page
2.6	Technical requirements	Describe the required software and hardware systems (if any).	0.5 page

ANNEX 8C. SELECTION CRITERIA MATRIX

Purpose: This Selection Criteria Matrix assists governments with the selection of a partner for outsourcing telemedicine or health hotline services (that is, when the government does not operate the service).

Timing: The matrix should be completed once potential partners have submitted proposals or quotations and before selecting a partner.

Instructions: Rank each of the criteria on a standard scale of 1–4 (except cost of work, which has a scale of 1–3), and then sum the total score for each potential partner. This method also allows for comparison and evaluation of the potential partners as well as identification of any strengths or weaknesses that may affect the overall decision.

CRITERIA	RANKING	SCORE
Strength of proposal		
Company background, including prior experience in implementing telemedicine or health hotline services	1 = No prior experience	
	2 = Limited prior experience for some parts of the scope of work	
	3 = Significant prior experience for at least some parts of the scope of work	
	4 = Significant experience for all aspects of the scope of work	
Prior experience working in-country or in similar country context	1 = No prior experience	
	2 = Limited experience in similar country	
	3 = Significant experience in similar country or limited experience in-country	
	4 = Significant prior experience working in-country	
Completeness of application (financial and compliance)	1 = Limited completeness of financial information and compliance-related information	
	2 = Moderate completeness of financial and compliance-related information	
	3 = Complete financial and compliance-related information	
	4 = Complete and favorable financial and compliance-related information	
Proposed approach or work plan	1 = Incomplete work plan that does not meet all project requirements	
	2 = Complete work plan that meets some but not all project requirements	
	3 = Complete work plan that meets all project requirements but is beyond the acceptable time frame for the project or does not represent a strong understanding of a project component (for example, is missing stakeholder engagement components)	
	4 = Complete work plan that meets all project requirements and meets timing requirements; suggests a strong understanding of all project components, such as governance, technology, and sustainability	

continued

CRITERIA	RANKING	SCORE
Relationship with partner		
Prior work with the partner	1 = Partner has previously been awarded contracts and has delivered subpar projects or demonstrated limitations in ability to manage projects	
	2 = Partner was previously unknown	
	3 = Partner has previously been awarded contracts and completed work satisfactorily	
	4 = Partner has previously been awarded contracts and has completed work projects in a timely fashion and produced high-quality output	
Cost		
Cost of work	1 = Cost far exceeds budget or seems unrealistic for project scope	
	2 = Cost is outside budget envelope	
	3 = Cost is within budget tolerance	
Total score		

NOTES

1. Numbeo, "Africa: Price Rankings by Country of Internet" (https://www.numbeo.com/cost-of-living/country_price_rankings?displayCurrency=USD&itemId=33&region=002).
2. Gartner Glossary, Information Technology Glossary, "Scalability" (https://www.gartner.com/en/information-technology/glossary/scalability).
3. Cisco, "What Is Cybersecurity" (https://www.cisco.com/c/en/us/products/security/what-is-cybersecurity.html).
4. For more information, see the Malawi Communications Regulatory Authority web page "Acts" (https://macra.mw/acts/).
5. For more information on FHIR (Fast Health Interoperability Resources), visit the HL7 International web page on this specification (https://fhir.org).
6. For more information, see SNOMED International (https://www.snomed.org); the World Health Organization's ICD (International Statistical Classification of Diseases and Related Health Problems) homepage (https://www.who.int/standards/classifications/classification-of-diseases); and the LOINC (Logical Observation Identifiers Names and Codes) home page (https://loinc.org).
7. For more information, visit the OpenHIE website (https://ohie.org/).

9

Cost and Validate the Five-Year Strategy and One-Year Road Map

Chapter 9 helps governments understand how to cost a telemedicine or health hotline service using all the outputs it has completed from Phase 2. Finally, after assessing preliminary costs, the government can validate the five-year strategy, one-year road map, and budget. This chapter presents the following tool:

- *Telemedicine or Health Hotline Cost Model Tool (annex 9A)*

COST THE SOLUTION FOR THE FIVE-YEAR STRATEGY AND ONE-YEAR ROAD MAP

The Telemedicine or Health Hotline Cost Model Tool in annex 9A estimates the cost associated with the government's preferred solution design. After analyzing potential costs, the government may need to modify these preferences to obtain a solution that fits its financial resources. The government uses the information from the responses to its requests for proposals or quotations for the preliminary costs, but it can do a final cost once it selects and contracts with a service provider (if applicable) in Phase 4. Additionally, if the government chooses to outsource, it can use this tool to understand necessary service provider costs to negotiate with the service provider.

The customizable Cost Model Tool estimates both start-up and ongoing costs. It integrates costing best practices for implementation, operation, and sustainability using VillageReach's previous experience with Chipatala Cha Pa Foni, or Health Center by Phone, in Malawi and with other partners to deliver more accurate estimates. Because the parameters used for this tool, such as unit costs, personnel salaries, and assumptions, are based on the solution in Malawi, they will need to be adjusted to specific country and solution contexts. The Cost Model Tool consists of the following key outputs:

- Estimate of start-up costs
- Estimate of ongoing operating and upgradation costs
- Estimate of the number of hotline workers needed
- Comparison of different options by cost

Methodology

To use the Cost Model Tool, the government will need the following information:

- Outputs of the five-year strategy regarding solution management (in-house versus outsourced), health areas, services, and geographic coverage
- Assumptions on the demand for the solution (for example, total expected call volume) and the target service level that should be included in any request for proposal or quotation
- Cost inputs from private sector firms using the requests for proposals or quotations, with the model assuming a "cost per hour of outsourcing call center," which will need to be compared to specific market rates (private sector) or salary ranges (public sector) in each country

If the government has this information readily available, completing the Cost Model Tool should take less than one hour. Several iterations of the tool will be required to test the cost of different scenarios—that is, the different unique mixes of service levels, health areas, technology types, and solution management (in-house versus outsourced) choices. Using the Cost Model Tool allows governments to develop different cost scenarios for potential funding requests.

Limitations of the cost model

The Cost Model Tool is important for estimating solution costs, but it also has four limitations:

1. *Nonexhaustive parameters:* Although built on a context applicable to many countries, the Cost Model Tool may lack certain parameters that could influence cost drivers in other countries. For example, the parameters do not include the socioeconomic situation of callers, because that information either was insignificant in the Malawi context or could not be accurately captured because of user protection regulations.

2. *User habits:* How users interact with the solution technology will affect solution costs, including user preferences for speaking with a health worker versus chatting through Short Message Service or WhatsApp, the length of interactions, and the complexity of the questions. User habits will vary from country to country and influence call or messaging volume. Although governments can adjust the Cost Model Tool to customize parameters to fit the local context, experience in that context will be required to get a more accurate picture.

3. *Cost optimization effect or impact:* The Cost Model Tool does not cover solution cost optimization over time.

4. *Total system effects:* The total cost of the services can change significantly depending on the strength of a country's health system and the level of involvement of private sector partners. Private sector involvement can significantly influence overall costs and can be more cost-effective in many cases. For example, creating agreements with mobile network operators to zero-rate calls can alleviate the otherwise high costs of calls. Additionally, some countries' health systems may have existing resources, both material and human, that can be used to support the service, thereby reducing overall costs.

VALIDATE FIVE-YEAR STRATEGY, ONE-YEAR ROAD MAP, AND PRELIMINARY COSTS/BUDGET

Once the focal point and planning task force have completed all the information gathering and preliminary costs, the government should hold another steering committee session to validate the five-year strategy, one-year road map, and preliminary costs. Depending on what the focal point presents for the costing, the strategy and road map may require some changes. Therefore, the final validation may take several steering committee meetings, as well as meeting with individual members. The focal point and planning task force should share findings in advance of steering committee meetings to help ensure alignment.

ANNEX 9A. TELEMEDICINE OR HEALTH HOTLINE COST MODEL TOOL

Purpose: The Telemedicine or Health Hotline Cost Model Tool (https://thedocs .worldbank.org/en/doc/171067ec8fb7059e81e748392e6406d3-0390012022 /original/5B-Telemedicine-Health-Hotline-Cost-Model-WB.xlsx) helps service providers estimate the costs of the solution associated with country context and country preferences.

Timing: This tool should be completed after gathering the outputs of the five-year strategy and one-year road map.

Instructions: Use the Excel file (https://thedocs.worldbank.org/en/doc /171067ec8fb7059e81e748392e6406d3-0390012022/original/5B-Telemedicine -Health-Hotline-Cost-Model-WB.xlsx). Instructions are on the first tab, and each tab has a different set of inputs.

Entering inputs

Mandatory inputs: The tool has two types of mandatory inputs, namely country context and country preferences, both of which significantly affect the overall cost of implementing and operating a telemedicine or health hotline.

Country context inputs include the following:

- Country name
- Population size
- Annual population growth rate
- Geographical scale to be covered (whole country, provinces, or districts)
- Population size of the scale to be covered
- Size of the scale to be covered
- Population aged 15–29 years of the scale to be covered
- Pregnant women of the scale to be covered
- Mobile network operator subscribers of the scale to be covered
- Active internet users of the scale to be covered
- Epidemic situation of the scale to be covered

All fields are mandatory. When the input cell has an in-cell drop-down option, please select input from the drop-down list.

Country preferences inputs include the following:

- Health topics to be covered
- Target population coverage for each health topic
- Technology to be used
- Target service level
- Operations/solution management

Predefined inputs: So that users can customize the cost model on a country-by-country basis, the Excel file lists separately many parameters and coefficients defined from the Chipatala Cha Pa Foni, or Health Center by Phone, experience in Malawi. The model will be able to correctly estimate the costs of different choices without manually filling in these inputs, but its accuracy can be greatly improved by modifying these values appropriately, because most of these values vary from country to country. These inputs are defined in three categories:

1. Personnel cost
2. Unit cost
3. Cost parameters

It is possible that the service, government, or other private sector partners will provide certain elements for free, such as the vehicle, the facility, or telecommunication services. It is possible that the government does not decide on certain elements, such as the vehicle or the generator. Please make sure that the unit cost of these cost elements is zero.

Unless necessary, kindly do not change the cost parameters (because without a good understanding of the calculation method used in the model, even small corrections can significantly change the cost model output).

Viewing the results

The cost estimate is divided into three main categories:

1. Start-up costs
2. Ongoing costs
3. Technical assistance costs

The cost model output provides the overall cost and the staffing required for the solution (estimate based on the Chipatala Cha Pa Foni experience in Malawi).

Comparing in-house and outsourced services costs

This cost model helps users choose the most cost-effective operations management by comparing in-house and outsourced services using the metric cost per productive time of an agent.

## 10

Conclusion: Next Steps

The validation of the five-year strategy, one-year road map, and preliminary costs marks the end of Phase 2. To ensure that it does not lose momentum, the government should consider the following steps in Phase 3 to solicit funding for start-up costs:

1. Allocate dedicated funding for telemedicine or health hotline services as part of the government's planning and budgeting cycle.
2. Competitively select partners and develop contracts.
3. Develop a service-level agreement using the Service-Level Agreement Tutorial in annex 10A.
4. Set up implementation plans using the Implementation and Planning for Sustainability from the Outset Checklist in annex 10B.
5. Continue to update steering committee members.
6. Begin implementing or stewarding the services.

One of the best ways for governments to learn about best practices, challenges, and sustainable approaches to establishing telemedicine or health hotline services is to talk to other governments that have gone through the process. Additionally, visiting any existing service centers to see how they are managed can be incredibly valuable for interested governments. For more information on the materials in this toolkit, or on connections to governments and service providers successfully managing these services, do not hesitate to reach out to the authors.

ANNEX 10A. SERVICE-LEVEL AGREEMENT TUTORIAL

Purpose: The Service-Level Agreement Tutorial (https://thedocs.worldbank .org/en/doc/9ee7ff265c220daffa8f3d61a3f9fa06-0390012022/original/6A -Service-Level-Agreement-Tutorial.pptx) explains the differences between a service-level agreement (SLA) and a contract, and it provides a high-level outline of what sections should be included in an SLA with a service provider. Because every government's template will be different, this outline is intended to provide general guidance.

Timing: The ministry of health will develop the SLA once it has secured funding (Phase 3) and is ready to contract with a service provider.

Instructions: The appropriate ministry of health department that has overall oversight for designing, implementing, and operating the solution will work with the partner to develop the SLA on the basis of the agreed technology, services, and scope identified during the strategy, road map, and costing validation process. The SLA generally includes the following elements:

- Statement of intent
- Scope
- Metrics and performance monitoring
- Planning and governance
- Deviations from standard processes and SLA
- Escalation and issue resolution
- Signatures

ANNEX 10B. IMPLEMENTATION AND PLANNING FOR SUSTAINABILITY FROM THE OUTSET CHECKLIST

Purpose: The Implementation and Planning for Sustainability from the Outset Checklist provides the government with guiding questions on how to begin planning with the selected partner for initial implementation of the telemedicine or hotline services. This planning would be done with scale and sustainability in mind from the beginning. Detailed implementation plans should be developed quickly after.

Timing: This table should be completed after the government has

- Selected a service provider and
- Established a preliminary contract.

Instructions: This checklist should be filled out by the government program manager together with the service provider program manager. Many of these items should already have been completed in the initial design, planning, and strategy; this checklist offers a chance to check on each step. Click "Yes," "No," or "n.a." (not applicable). The use of "Yes"/"No" is meant to make sure the service provider does not forget any critical conversations or items. Rather than an extensive plan, the checklist is a tool to guide planning for sustainability from the outset. For any "No" response, develop action points for addressing these items in the planning tools.

#	STRATEGIC AREA	GUIDING QUESTIONS	YES/NO/N.A.
1	Identifying key counterparts and approach	Have you identified the decision-making focal point within the government?	❑ Yes ❑ No ❑ n.a.
		Has the government identified any additional on-the-ground partners (implementing/private) needed to implement and operate the solution in the long run?	❑ Yes ❑ No ❑ n.a.
		Has the government identified any additional private sector or other partners that might implement different elements of the solution aside from the primary implementer (for example, for added capabilities—WhatsApp or interactive voice response)?	❑ Yes ❑ No ❑ n.a.
		Has the government established other relationships needed to negotiate competitive ongoing costs for the government (for example, with mobile network operators)?	❑ Yes ❑ No ❑ n.a.
		Has the partner/government/funder identified how the solution will be run and paid for in the long run?	❑ Yes ❑ No ❑ n.a.
2	Stakeholder alignment	Have the partners discussed roles and responsibilities of the different partners?	❑ Yes ❑ No ❑ n.a.
		Is there documented agreement by all partners on roles and responsibilities (in the form of a signed letter, memorandum of understanding, signed plan, RACI [responsible, accountable, consulted, and informed] chart, or the like)?	❑ Yes ❑ No ❑ n.a.
		Has everyone agreed on the data-sharing stipulations and monitoring and evaluation indicators? (See the monitoring and evaluation section of this tool for details.)	❑ Yes ❑ No ❑ n.a.
		Does the government have a technical working group or other network of stakeholders to work with to drive forward implementation and decision-making? (Note: Having such a group will also help with sustainability planning.)	❑ Yes ❑ No ❑ n.a.
3	Formative assessment	Have there been discussions with key in-country stakeholders and partners on how the existing solution will be adapted to fit the government's specific needs? Consider specific areas for potential adaptation around the following:	❑ Yes ❑ No ❑ n.a.
		Solution design—for example, does the solution have elements that need to be adjusted for given the technical design needed?	❑ Yes ❑ No ❑ n.a.
		Community engagement/sensitization	❑ Yes ❑ No ❑ n.a.
		Resource availability	❑ Yes ❑ No ❑ n.a.
		Financial management	❑ Yes ❑ No ❑ n.a.
		Government strategic alignment	❑ Yes ❑ No ❑ n.a.
		Policy and regulation	❑ Yes ❑ No ❑ n.a.

continued

#	STRATEGIC AREA	GUIDING QUESTIONS	YES/NO/N.A.
4	Solution description	Is the solution documented in a format accessible to all relevant stakeholders in the receiving country?	❏ Yes ❏ No ❏ n.a.
		Has the solution been adapted to fit the specific needs and context of the country according to the formative assessment?	❏ Yes ❏ No ❏ n.a.
		If not, is there a plan for what needs to be done to adapt it (needs, plan, and resources)?	❏ Yes ❏ No ❏ n.a.
5	Resource availability	Have the partners agreed what level of personnel is needed to manage and operate the solution?	❏ Yes ❏ No ❏ NA
		If the plan is to eventually embed the actual operation into government systems, do the jobs and positions needed for this solution exist in the government's current, established human resource list?	❏ Yes ❏ No ❏ n.a.
		If the plan is to embed operations but the jobs and positions do not exist in the established human resource list, is it known what the plan would be to get them added in the long run?	❏ Yes ❏ No ❏ n.a.
		Do the people who will operate, maintain, and evaluate the solution have the skills required?	❏ Yes ❏ No ❏ n.a.
		If the government will eventually operate the service, does the government or partner have the buildings, equipment, and technology (if applicable) necessary to manage and operate the solution?	❏ Yes ❏ No ❏ n.a.
6	Financial management	Have projected solution costs for startup been updated according to the final solution's functional and technical design as determined with the service provider?	❏ Yes ❏ No ❏ n.a.
		Have projected solution costs for scaling been updated?	❏ Yes ❏ No ❏ n.a.
		Have projected solution costs for ongoing implementation been updated according to the government's specific needs, its context, and elements the government has decided to move forward?	❏ Yes ❏ No ❏ n.a.
		If real or potential funding gaps from government sources exist, is there a strategy in place to cover funding gaps?	❏ Yes ❏ No ❏ n.a.
		If the government will take over direct payment in the long term, does it have the necessary mechanisms in place to disburse funds and to contract, as needed, for any elements it does not operate in-house?	❏ Yes ❏ No ❏ n.a.

continued

#	STRATEGIC AREA	GUIDING QUESTIONS	YES/NO/N.A.
7	Government strategy	Are there people in all relevant national ministries who will generate interest for the adoption and implementation of the solution?	❑ Yes ❑ No ❑ n.a.
		Is the government decentralized?	❑ Yes ❑ No ❑ n.a.
		If so, does the solution require different government representatives at multiple levels for budgeting, adoption, advertising, and implementation? Discuss who these people are.	❑ Yes ❑ No ❑ n.a.
		Does the government have a health strategy, and is this type of solution specifically addressed in that health strategy?	❑ Yes ❑ No ❑ n.a.
8	Policy and regulation	Are new laws and policies needed to support the telemedicine or health hotline solution implementation and management?	❑ Yes ❑ No ❑ n.a.
		Is the solution compatible with existing laws and policies?	❑ Yes ❑ No ❑ n.a.
		If not, is it possible or desirable to advocate for changes in laws and policies? (If not, replication should be reconsidered.)	❑ Yes ❑ No ❑ n.a.
9	Organization	Has the government considered what effective governance structures for solution management and operation are needed within this country and context?	❑ Yes ❑ No ❑ n.a.
10	Monitoring and evaluation alignment	Are targets clearly articulated and agreed upon in writing by stakeholders?	❑ Yes ❑ No ❑ n.a.
		Do the indicators need to be rolled into specific reporting standards or systems (for example, District Health Information Software or other systems)?	❑ Yes ❑ No ❑ n.a.
		Is the ability to capture that information already available?	❑ Yes ❑ No ❑ n.a.
	Total Yes:		
	Total No:		
	Total n.a.:		

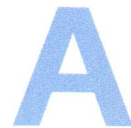

Checklist of Challenges and Pitfalls That May Arise during Planning or Implementing Telemedicine or Health Hotline Services, and Potential Mitigating Actions

Background: This checklist is derived from real experiences and background research on telemedicine or health hotline services implementation. Although not an exhaustive list, it may help governments from the outset. Additionally, many of the chapters in the toolkit are designed to help governments address potential challenges before they become real challenges.

POTENTIAL CHALLENGES AND PITFALLS	POTENTIAL MITIGATING ACTIONS
Governance challenges	
Lack of clear decision-making	Establish strong governance at the project outset (see toolkit chapters 3 and 5), both within the government and with any external stakeholders. Governments need to ensure from the beginning that ministries of health identify which department will operate the solution. For each solution decision, such as spending funds or selecting a technology vendor, continue to empower the proper governance body and ultimate decision-maker with each project milestone. Document all decisions. Additionally, to ensure continuity, ensure that decision-making lies within a position's job description rather than relying on an individual person.
Multiple silos or competing services	Collaborate and coordinate with existing partners and services. When possible, build on what exists. Create a governance mechanism for coordinating services to avoid overlap (see the section in chapter 4 titled "Design high-level solution"). Help partners understand that everyone is working toward the same goal: to improve the country's health outcomes.
Challenges related to mobile network operators	
Challenges with zero-rating calls by mobile network operators (MNOs)	Gaining MNO commitment and follow-through for zero-rate calls can be challenging. The government should be clear whether it seeks an optional commitment by the MNO or will institute a government regulatory action or requirement. Document commitments and expectations along the way. Use high-level officials to have the conversations with the MNO managing directors. Explain how zero-rate calls will benefit the MNO.

continued

POTENTIAL CHALLENGES AND PITFALLS	POTENTIAL MITIGATING ACTIONS
Challenges with MNO interoperability	Having MNOs route calls or short codes to a telemedicine or health hotline service is important but can be challenging. Establish memorandums of understanding or up-front commitments on how to work with each MNO, and document commitments along the way.
Challenges with MNOs requiring exclusivity agreements	An MNO may want to have exclusivity for three or more years. Negotiate early if it is critical that the services connect through multiple mobile networks. If needed, the government may agree to the exclusivity agreement but should make sure to build an end date into any memorandums of understanding.
Technology challenges	
Hotline and technology capacity	The number of callers can exceed telemedicine or health hotline staff capacity or the technology limits (for example, the number of lines). Plan for expected capacity up front, and regularly track ongoing use. Every call center, hotline, or telemedicine service must constantly manage supply and demand by changing staffing levels or schedules and changing how and when the service is promoted.
Program management challenges	
Timeline delays	As with any multistakeholder or technology project, it is easy for timelines to shift. Establish clear expectations between stakeholders, create a project timeline with key milestones, and meet regularly to review progress. Identify delays or deviations, and discuss a course of action to get back on track. For any contracted service provider, build a strong service-level agreement or contract with clear deliverables, and hold the service providers to those deliverables before paying them.
Financing challenges	
Initial funding runs out	Many telemedicine or health hotline services have ended when the social impact organization runs out of donor funding for the program. A government needs to include financing for these services within its strategic planning and budgeting exercise and have clear plans that estimate both start-up and ongoing costs from the beginning. Through the steering committee, look at multiple avenues of sustaining the service long term. The telemedicine or health hotline services could help with universal health coverage across departments, including the services in the strategic plans and budgets to advocate within the government. Also consider adding a small budget line from each relevant department in the ministry of health to maintain the cost of the service. If the service is set up in-house, the goal should be to establish it as its own unit (or combine it with another relevant unit, like emergency medicine) with its own budget to ensure it always has a place in future ministry of health budgets.

B

PowerPoint Template for Pitching Telemedicine or Health Hotline Services to Governments

Background: High-level government officials like to understand what problem is being addressed, what a solution entails, expected outcomes (the health impact), costs (when possible), and next steps. This PowerPoint (https://thedocs .worldbank.org/en/doc/e452cf2c0b46d1e4076fd3b9e9822ba0-0390012023 /original/Appendix-B-PowerPoint-Template-for-pitching-telemedicine -health-hotline-services-to-governments.pptx) serves as a template based on an example of what was presented to several different governments. It can be adapted as needed to fit the context.

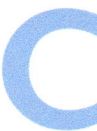

VillageReach and Praekelt.org Sample Health Hotline and Messaging Service Pitch to a Ministry of Health

---

Background: This PDF (https://thedocs.worldbank.org/en/doc/1b4f29ad2 e2c7b0057449c0fcaad3efb-0390012023/original/11-3-Appendix-C -VillageReach-Praekelt-org-example-Health-Hotline-and-Messaging-Service -Pitch-to-MOH.pdf) provides an example of a pitch deck presented to a ministry of health in Sub-Saharan Africa to show the potential for providing public nationwide health hotline and messaging services in the country.

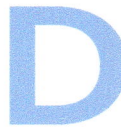

Sample Implementation Toolkit from Malawi's Chipatala Cha Pa Foni

Background: VillageReach created the Chipatala Cha Pa Foni (CCPF), or Health Center by Phone, Toolkit (https://thedocs.worldbank.org/en/doc /8878ea19d150e4f5a8cf956a513876cd-0390012023/original/Appendix-D -Example-Implementation-Toolkit-from-Malawi-HCBP.pdf) in collaboration with and for the Malawi Ministry of Health as part of solution transition. This toolkit provides the Ministry of Health with materials needed to operate and manage CCPF. It is divided into eight main sections, with two additional sections for appendixes and annexes. It has several standard operating procedures that could be used and adapted in any setting. Each main section has its own corresponding appendixes section. Electronic links are provided for both the main and appendixes section. Although this toolkit is specific to the CCPF in Malawi, it still provides governments with an understanding of what they need for ongoing implementation and management of the services and can be adapted to meet specific country needs. Note that in the Malawi model the government is the owner and manager. CCPF is operated in-house, though the government does contract with a service provider to maintain the software and has an agreement with Airtel, the mobile network operator, to zero-rate the calls.

The main standard operating procedures of the toolkit are available in PDF, but the related appendixes and tools are on the Trello board here: https://trello .com/invite/b/P77JLFJf/4e009c1278aa1adb09c66a3fccc4a6f5/chipatala -cha-pa-foni-ccpf. It is open to anyone, but users must register first. The QR code is also available below:

Understanding Regulatory Prerequisites Reference Materials

For many private sector firms providing equipment or software for public health solutions, there are no regulatory prerequisites, unless the technology will capture, store, or transmit patient data. For situations in which the government fully outsources telemedicine or health hotline services to an external firm or call center, it is important that regulations for both quality of care and customer/patient information management are clearly defined. In addition to being critical for a patient's well-being, these regulatory topics provide a definable operating environment, which is important for private sector firms to define, implement, and operate sustainable business operations. In the absence of regulatory clarity, private sector firms may hesitate to provide services or may invest only minimally without more certainty around the regulatory prerequisites. Development of these regulatory documents is out of scope for this toolkit.

Some countries have developed standards that can be used as references. For example, the Health Professions Council of South Africa has developed the "General Ethical Guidelines for Good Practice in Telemedicine" (https://www.sada.co.za/media/documents/HPCSA_Booklet_10_Telemedicine.pdf), and here is an example of a practice guideline (https://www.cno.org/globalassets/docs/prac/41041_telephone.pdf) from Ontario (CNO 2020; HPCSA 2014).

REFERENCES

CNO (College of Nurses of Ontario). 2020. *Telepractice*. Practice Guideline. Toronto: CNO. https://www.cno.org/globalassets/docs/prac/41041_telephone.pdf.

HPCSA (Health Professions Council of South Africa). 2014. "General Ethical Guidelines for Good Practice in Telemedicine." Booklet No. 10, HPCSA, Pretoria. https://www.sada.co.za/media/documents/HPCSA_Booklet_10_Telemedicine.pdf.